What We See and What We Say

Image-based research methods, such as arts-based research, can fill the absence of the voice of impoverished, under-privileged populations. In *What We See and What We Say*, Ephrat Huss argues that images are deep and universally psycho-neurological constructs through which people process their experiences. The theoretical model demonstrated in this book demonstrates that images can be used to enable three different levels of communication: with self, with others similar to oneself, and with others who differ in terms of culture and power. Dr. Huss centers her argument on a case study of impoverished Bedouin women's groups in Israel who used art as self-expression, and includes many additional examples such as unemployed women and teenage girls in slums, women who underwent sexual abuse, and the experiences of illegal immigrants. Ultimately, the author points to how the inherent structural characteristics of images help to intensify the voices of marginalized groups in research, therapy, empowerment, and social action.

Ephrat Huss, PhD, is an art therapist, a social worker, and a senior lecturer and founder of the Arts in Social Work Masters Specialization at the Charlotte B. and Jack J. Spirtzer Department of Social Work at Ben-Gurion University of the Negev in Israel.

What We See and What We Say
Using Images in Research, Therapy, Empowerment, and Social Change

Ephrat Huss

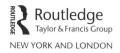

NEW YORK AND LONDON

First published 2013
by Routledge
711 Third Avenue, New York, NY 10017

Simultaneously published in the UK
by Routledge
27 Church Road, Hove, East Sussex BN3 2FA

Routledge is an imprint of the Taylor & Francis Group, an informa business

© 2013 Taylor & Francis

The right of Ephrat Huss to be identified as author of this work has been asserted by her in accordance with sections 77 and 78 of the Copyright, Designs and Patents Act 1988.

All rights reserved. No part of this book may be reprinted or reproduced or utilised in any form or by any electronic, mechanical, or other means, now known or hereafter invented, including photocopying and recording, or in any information storage or retrieval system, without permission in writing from the publishers.

Trademark notice: Product or corporate names may be trademarks or registered trademarks, and are used only for identification and explanation without intent to infringe.

Library of Congress Cataloging in Publication Data
Huss, Ephrat.
　What we see and what we say : using images in research, therapy, empowerment, and social change / by Ephrat Huss. — 1st ed.
　p. cm.
　1. Visual sociology—Research. 2. Social change. I. Title.
　HM500.H87 2013
　303.4—dc23
　　　　　　　　　　　　　　　　　　　　　　　　2012026483

ISBN: 978-0-415-51035-6 (hbk)
ISBN: 978-0-203-12434-5 (ebk)

Typeset in Sabon
by EvS Communication Networx, Inc.

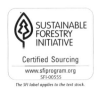

Printed and bound in the United States of America by
Walsworth Publishing Company, Marceline, MO.

Contents

Acknowledgments vii

Introduction 1

SECTION 1
Art as a Speech Act from the Margins: A Case Study of Impoverished Bedouin Women's Images 9

1 Social Context: Background to the Bedouin Women's Case Study 11

2 Working with Images: The Method Used in the Case Study 19

3 Bedouin Women's Images on the Level of Content 26

4 Pain and Resilience as Seen in the Compositional Elements of the Bedouin Women's Images 38

SECTION 2
Using Images from a Socially Contextualized Perspective within Social Research and Practice 49

5 Using Images in Research from a Social Perspective 51

   Figure Section

6 Methodological Implications of Using Images within Research 63

7 Art Therapy: The Missing Social Theory of Art Therapy 73

8 Methodology of a Socially Contextualized Art Therapy	85
9 Images as Group Empowerment and Action	94
10 Images in Conflict Negotiation with Power Holders	103
11 Summary	113
Bibliography	115
Index	128

Acknowledgments

For Boaz, my husband, whose love is my support and inspiration.

I would like to give deep thanks to Professor Julie Cwikel, who supervised my "strange" visual doctoral project with Bedouin women—who believed in me—and who relentlessly demanded that I translate my visual insights into the highest standard of academic writing. Thank you.

A special thanks for the grant provided by the Robert H. Arnow Center for Bedouin Studies and Development: Ben Gurion University that enabled me to undertake my doctoral research that is the base of the central case study of this book.

Introduction

Each morning, as the dramas of my dreams are still with me, the Muezzin's call to prayer enters my bedroom. The source of that rising and falling voice, a Bedouin village less than 5 kilometers from my home, is nowhere to be seen. Surrounding my house are the other red-roofed homes of a Jewish settlement, shrouded in bright green foliage that keeps the desert out. What I see and what I hear tell me different stories, but together these stories create a multifaceted narrative. Over the course of this project, I held image-based workshops, which were designed to illustrate the use of images in social theory and practice, with impoverished Bedouin women in the basements of buildings or in huts. Despite their dilapidated condition, the buildings where women's groups are held are a change from the pervasive poverty the Bedouin women endure; ironically, in these shabby buildings are enrichment opportunities: literacy classes, computer courses, driving lessons, lectures on rights and health, and arts workshops, such as the one I organized.

Since the beginning of my research, I have gotten to know some of the buildings and some of the women in the Bedouin village next to the Jewish settlement where I live in the southern desert region of Israel; women who remain out of view and whose voices are not heard over the Muezzin's loud speakers. Our weekly sessions together are vivid in memory, most especially the ways that the images that we explored enabled me to learn about their and my own pain, as well as their resilience, their ability to cope, and the constant negotiation of a meeting point between individual and social experience.

On the days we were lucky, the old fan whirled, bringing a respite from the intense heat. The room at times reverberated with lively stories about the women's drawings, resulting in emotional closeness; at other times silence filled the room. How does the joint construction and explanation of images impact the relationship between images and words, as well as the relationship between the marginalized Bedouin women in the huts and myself, a Jewish middle-class researcher? When I suggested that we summarize the meaning of these crafts and drawing sessions, the women nodded their heads politely and thanked me, ignoring my questions. The aim of this book is to demonstrate the process of creating images and crafts, discussing them, and showing them to similar and different participants. Implications of this process will be connected to social practice and theory, demonstrating how images can unite research, therapy, empowerment, conflict negotiation, and social action into a joint, underlying theory for utilizing images from a social perspective.

These workshops taught me how images can simultaneously serve as data, therapy, empowerment, and a vehicle for social change and dialogue with power holders from different cultures. Images were shown to be informative as well as transformative on different levels. The creation of images enabled the women to concretely map out spaces that had been taken away from them, as well as to symbolize, and thus explore, their pain. These images also revealed how the women cope and negotiate their needs. How do images enable these multiple and synergetic roles?

Humans are wired to respond emotionally to the sight of images. The psychological response that is triggered translates composition into meaningful content and connects this information with emotional arousal. Images are thus a central axis for connecting senses, cognition, and emotion (Conway, 2009; Nelson & Fivush, 2004; Sarid & Huss 2010). On a universal level, images are a deep psychoneurological construct through which people process their experiences. Being central to human functioning, images contribute to an individual's ability to remain oriented in the world by retaining memories of past experiences and providing a means of problem-solving based on these preserved images. For example, the ability to quickly differentiate a dangerous object (such as a tiger) as distinct from its background and to generate emotional arousal from this information enables survival.

Image construction undergoes universal stages of development that parallel our cognitive ability to begin to think in more abstract terms. From a developmental perspective, the ability to process images matures before the ability to process words and influences the ability to connect abstract symbols, such as words, to images that have also become schematized (Mathews, 1994; Williams & Wood, 1984).

Diagnostic use of images by social practitioners aims to assess stress and development and is based on universal developmental stages. The projective characteristics of images reveal unconscious feelings and defenses, according to dynamic psychological theories (Silver, 2005). Jung points to universal images as symbols or archetypes that can be found in different variations in all cultures (Jung, 1974).

On the other hand, Gardner (1993) suggests that images are not universal but are socially constructed. He points to the dominance of different types of discrete intelligences—visual, verbal, audio, and kinetic—within individuals, as well as within different cultures. Gardner claims, for example, that Western culture predominates in verbal and mathematical skills, while in nomadic cultures, for example, kinesthetic and visual skills predominate (Gardner, 1993). Thus, from a cultural perspective, while image formation undergoes set stages of development, different aesthetic norms are imparted within this process due to cultural influences. For example, in traditional cultures, exactitude and aesthetics are important from a very early age, while, in Western cultures, individualized emotional self-expression and individualistic values are important from an early age (Lowenfield, 1987).

We see that, on the one hand, images reflect the subjective experience of their creator; but, on the other hand, they are also constructed within a specific social and cultural context that defines their content and aesthetics. Because of this duality, images are created by, but also embody a reaction to the social norms that they represent (Mahon, 2000). From this perspective, aesthetics are expressions of, and dialogues with, socially specific rather than universal beliefs. Images show how people understand, experience, react to, and cope with, the social contexts that define them. This is what makes the study of images so useful for the social sciences.

We see that images can be described as a meeting point between cognitive and emotional understandings, as well as between universal, personal, and culturally constructed understandings. Images are always created within and defined by a specific social context, but they also express an individual's phenomenological experience of that social construct. For example, all teenage girls will doodle heart shapes, but these hearts will be differently constructed, placed, and explained within different social contexts and according to different girls; the scrawled or carefully constructed hearts thus constantly redefine a social reality. For example, within Bedouin embroidery, the heart shape has now been added as a symbol of love in the Western sense (Tal, 1980).

Therefore, the study of images can be understood as a means of revealing the connection between personal identity and society. This meeting place between the personal and the social underlines the deep relevance of exploring images and their construction in research areas such as education, sociology, geography, and anthropology, as well as for social practitioners such as psychologists, social workers, and educators.

Because all of these fields are based on language, the inclusion of images creates a dialogue between two different forms. Often images are used to illustrate, entertain, or distract, rather than as the central content or form within research or social practice. In contrast, a new relationship between images and words is sought within arts-based research in education, where images are utilized to ignite fresh perspectives on issues (Eisner, 1997). Visual anthropology and visual studies utilize visual constructs as a way to understand the cultures and systems that produce them (Emerson & Smith, 2000; Pink & Kurti, 2004).

In community art and in art as social change, images are used as a way to destabilize existing power structures (Butler, 2001; Harrington, 2004; Shank, 2005). The power structure between images and words is dynamic; images are sometimes understood as a more authentic or universal form of expression than words are, as in art therapy (Rose, 1988), or in humanistic perspectives and arts-based research (McNiff, 1995). Sullivan (2001) describes image making as an inherent type of "laboratory" or form of research in and of itself.

From this perspective, using images in research as illustrations for language is considered a reduction of their inherent characteristics. Alternatively, others claim that the relevance of images is that they can clarify or illustrate concepts and words (Bowler, 1997; Brington & Lykes, 1996; Foster, 2007; Simmons & Hicks, 2006; Wang & Burris, 1994).

In social practice, image-based methods such as guided imagery and art therapy are also rapidly expanding. Research points to the healing potential of arts to reestablish communication between mind and body and cognition and to transform painful memories into a more tolerable form (Chamberlan & Smith, 2008; Kaye & Bleep, 1997; Sarid & Huss, 2010; Warren, 2008).

Overall, the use of images in social science is different from their use in the fine arts. The social sciences are not focused on the quality of the product according to aesthetic standards but, rather, are focused on the product as a method to initiate explanation or impact society (Mullen, 2003). The image is understood in terms of process, product, and explanation, rather than as a discrete entity that is separate from its creator and is evaluated by critics. This distinction, however, is also blurred, as some movements in fine art, such as community-oriented art, also seek to become more communicative and relevant to society as a whole, by stepping out of the galleries into places that create social impact (Butler, 2001; Harrington, 2004; Shank, 2005).

We see that, although there is an explosion in image use in different fields of the social sciences, the underlying commonalities of using images based on their own inherent characteristics as a lateral perspective is lacking. The aim of this book is to demonstrate a common base or foundation of image use as a continuum for social researchers in different fields and for different types of social practitioners. This common base is explored within this book, so as to suggest a theoretical model for including visual images within research and practice in the social sciences based on the characteristics of images in synergy with the discrete fields that use them.

This book is divided into two sections; the first section is based upon an extended case study of the images made by marginalized Bedouin women in Israel. These images reveal social context but also reveal how people experience and cope within that context. This provides a method and analytical prism for understanding and implementing images through a social lens.

The second section of the book will reintegrate this prism into the central areas of social research and practice that utilize images, including arts-based research, art therapy, social empowerment, social change, and conflict negotiation. This section will be based on the Bedouin women's case study but will also include additional examples of images made by different groups of marginalized people, such as impoverished unemployed Jewish women in Israel and teenagers living in slums, as well as the images made by disaster survivors in Sri Lanka, but also populations such as survivors of sexual abuse or social workers and art therapy students.

A description of each chapter in the book follows:

Section 1: Art as a Speech Act from the Margins: A Case Study of Impoverished Bedouin Women's Images

The first chapter will outline the social context of the impoverished Bedouin women whose images will be presented in this study. This chapter will discuss the intersecting oppressions of gender, culture, and poverty for a community undergoing rapid transition from a nomadic, collective society to a sedentary, individualistic one. This context is made relevant for other marginalized and impoverished groups that experience immigration, globalization, or urbanization.

The transition from traditional to Western or from collective to individual or from nomadic to sedentary culture will be defined in terms of its impact on gender roles and also on the types of images that women create and have access to. The shifting roles of the women will be shown to be reflected in the shift of aesthetic and symbolic mechanisms within the cultural images of the Bedouin women and in the creation of new and hybrid cultural aesthetics.

In the second chapter, the method of the case study will be outlined, integrating a phenomenological and social theoretical prism. This method aims to understand images as simultaneously a construct of, but also a reaction to, social and cultural reality, and as a tool to change that reality.

The field method, the ethics, and the analytical prism used in the case study will be outlined as exemplifying central dilemmas of including images from a socially contextualized perspective in research and practice, such as who defines the image, process, and meaning of the image. These dilemmas will be further explored throughout the book.

The third chapter will present a thematic analysis of the images themselves, focusing on the content of the Bedouin women's images as explained by them. These images in the symbolic and concrete space of the page reveal their needs—mobility, houses, outside spaces, educational spaces—as well as their desire either to enter Western culture or to be protected by traditional culture. The level of poverty that the women experience leaves them with no resources to help them fully enter either cultural direction and thus, ultimately, leaves them with no spaces, either on the page or in reality. Mapping this lack of space will reveal the multiple levels of oppression the women endure, from both the Israeli state and the Bedouin patriarchy.

The fourth chapter will address the compositional aesthetic elements of these images, focusing on how the women symbolize their pain and define it as due to social oppression rather than due to inherent weakness. From this perspective, the compositional analysis does not reveal pathology, as in diagnostic tests, but rather illustrates strengths and coping, indirect resistance to oppression, and negotiation of power through symbols and metaphors. The images and their explanations will focus on the self-defined solutions of the women to their problems and will include the aesthetic strategies of integrating opposing cultural realities, resisting lack of spaces, and recreating a collective voice.

These in-depth analyses of the women's images show the social reality of the Bedouin women that constructs these images, as well as what these women feel and how they cope with the shifting social reality. This is another layer of construction within the images.

Section 2: Using Images from a Socially Contextualized Perspective within Social Research and Practice

In the second half of the book the theoretical and methodological principles that emerged from the first half of the book will be applied to the areas that use images within social sciences, such as arts-based research and visual culture, art therapy, group empowerment, and social action. The aim of this application is to show how these fields can integrate phenomenological and social analyses to not only access cultural reality, but also to interpret the experience of a culture, resulting in a base for individual, group, and social change.

Chapter 5 will address the uses of images in research. This chapter shows how social and phenomenological perspectives combine to enable images to challenge hegemonic verbal discourses, becoming relevant to indigenous feminist and action research. Images enable the capture of painful and taboo subjects that are projected onto, and distanced by, the use of images. The images will be shown to reveal a complex social reality but also to enable a meeting between cognitive (or socially accepted narratives) and emotional (or personal experience) narratives. The chapter will also show how images capture elusive information such as how people integrate opposing cultural understandings and negotiate social realities—on the level of showing rather than telling.

This is an additional prism for understanding images in researching hybrid cultural realities and marginal positions. The chapter points to how images can become a method for revealing how research participants self-define solutions to problems within complex and shifting situations. This method will be demonstrated with additional case studies.

The sixth chapter will continue the themes of the fifth chapter and aims to translate these theoretical implications into methodological implications for the use of images in research. This translation starts with addressing how images are defined, how the process of creating or choosing an image is conceived, and how the process of explaining an image is negotiated from a multiple perspective. These considerations are turned into a theoretical model that defines the position of images within research as method, data, subject, or object. The advantages and disadvantages of the placement of images as method, additional data, subject, object, or outcome of research are presented, with examples from additional research projects.

Chapter 7 will outline the implications of using a social prism for understanding and implementing images within art therapy. Socially critical art therapy, which is contextualized within culture and power relations, defines a problem and a solution as an expression in an image resulting from a social and cultural perspective. This is a missing theory within art therapy that tends to be based on dynamic or humanistic understandings of art as expressed from within.

Chapter 8 aims to address the method for using art therapy from this theoretical prism. This method challenges current definitions of process, images, and their analyses, as well as challenging the role and education of the art therapist. From this perspective, images are shown to ignite coping and resilience within a specific social context through integrating as well as questioning social norms that perpetuate the problem. Examples and additional case studies will be provided to illustrate this method; for example, a study that illustrates a model of art therapy that initially defines the social reality of a problem, and then continues to define the stress and coping reactions synergistically in relation to the problem, integrating context, stress reactions, and resiliences as seen within a single image.

Chapter 9 continues this social perspective from personal transformation in therapy into group empowerment models: This reveals how images create an individual space to critique or to transform a social narrative within a group of similar others; these dual symbolic spaces—the group and the image—will be shown with the help of different case studies, to enable new and integrated or coherent group narratives to be defined before turning to external power holders. If the two previous chapters on art therapy call for an inclusion of the social into the subjective, then this and the following chapter exemplify the contribution of the phenomenological or personal space to the social levels of using images to initiate social change.

Chapter 10 will show how images are integrated into social action and conflict negotiation, claiming that an image can be an effective space to create communication between different levels of power and different cultures and so be used to negotiate power within conflicted groups. Images are shown to be an indirect source of influence but still succeed in triggering emotions and eliciting empathy, and as such they are shown to be effective tools for communication with others. The use of images to create a more flextime type of transitional space between conflict groups, based on the above reasons, and on the ability of images to shift perspectives from political to phenomenological experience, still within a social context, are outlined with the help of additional case studies.

Section 1
Art as a Speech Act from the Margins
A Case Study of Impoverished Bedouin Women's Images

This section will provide the social context of the case study, and the research strategy and setting as background to understanding the images that will be presented and analyzed, first by the women themselves.

The images that the marginalized Bedouin women created in the study's workshops can be understood in terms of a social theoretical prism that will demonstrate the combined oppressive power of cultural transition, poverty, and gender discrimination for these women. The content of the images will be shown to express this social reality in a complex way, while the compositional elements will reveal how the women feel and cope with this reality. This includes pain, but also constant struggle against these oppressions. The discussion of the images will be shown to create a coherent group narrative and a way to indirectly influence and resist power holders.

1 Social Context
Background to the Bedouin Women's Case Study

This chapter will provide the social and research context of the case study of marginalized Bedouin women in Israel, who are used to exemplify the theory of this book. This chapter will also outline the social context of the impoverished Bedouin women in Israel, as well as the research strategy used to develop and organize the art workshops with them. This context is specific, yet also characteristic of other indigenous and transitioning impoverished women in the world. The research design described in this section aims to touch upon the problems or the issues that arise when using images within a research or empowerment setting.

A premise of this study is that social context cannot only be learned from textbooks as a static anthropological entity. Social context involves a hybridization of various—and at times conflicting—norms or cultural processes within any given person and group at any given time (Abu-Lughod, 1993; Avruch, 1998; Bhabha, 1994; Spindler, 1997). In accordance with this assumption a static description of traditional Bedouin culture, as described in the literature, will first be outlined, and then the cultural transition that this group underwent with the setting up of the state of Israel will be described.

A. Traditional Bedouin Culture and Collectivist Values

Although the Bedouin are Muslim, they have integrated early pre-Islamic customs into Islam, specifically those related to survival in the desert. The term *Bedouin* refers to the Arab nomadic tribes that have lived in Israel for over two millennia (Meir, 1997). Within the Negev, there are three types of Bedouin: the "Sum Ran," considered the original Bedouin tribes, the "El-Abed," who are black Sudanese Bedouin, and the "Hum Ran," who are Arab *fallachim* who joined the Bedouin tribes (Baily, 2002; Barakat, 1993; Meir, 1997).

The term *Bedouin* does not imply a unified racial, ethnic, or national group but rather refers to groups that reside in desert lands. These groups include a myriad of people with different degrees of sedantarization, agriculture, and nomadic lifestyles. Tribes are organized along political rather than racial lines (Meir, 1997; Relton, 2005).

In terms of social organization within traditional Bedouin culture, the concept of collectivism is a central component, as it is in most traditional rural cultures. Sue (1996) describes identity within collective societies as based on an outer locus of control, which means that identity is defined in terms of relationships within the family or tribe rather than in terms of personal achievement. According to Cole (1996), context is not the "surroundings" external to the individual, but rather the "connected whole that gives coherence to its parts" (Cole, 1996, p. 135).

Collectivist culture has been described as "the production of selves with fluid boundaries organized for gendered and aged domination" (Joseph, 1999, p. 12; Eidelman, 2002). Suad (1997) describes Arab patriarchal power as being central at familial, institutional, and public levels, with the extended family as the most central unit of Muslim society. Individual actions reflect upon the family as a whole and vice versa. The values of generosity, hospitality, reciprocity, pride, valor, and strength are manifested through societal codes of indirect communication, conflict avoidance, and the use of mediators (Cole, 1996; Joseph, 1999; Suad, 1997; Tal, 1980, 1995). Another way of defining these values is as "high context," according to Barakat (1993), emphasizing the collective over the individual, a slow pace of societal change, and a sense of social stability as a value.

B. Women Within Traditional Culture

Traditional cultures are gender segregated: Women often do not have access to legal assistance, cannot choose their husbands, and have no control over the family's finances, including their own dowries (Hijab, 1988). Within this traditional context, women establish power relative to other Bedouin women, not in the male public arena. Traditionally, women's social life and power are found in the home, rather than within public spaces, where their power is limited. The home, run by women, is lively and bustling, and it is an arena for working out different familial issues. Conversely, the men interact among themselves in public areas. Lewando-Hundt (1976, 1978) describes how the traditional Bedouin tent has designated women's areas, in which women's tasks such as childcare and cooking take place, and designated men's areas, where people from the outside are hosted and where decisions are made overtly. Traditionally, in situations of conflict negotiation, Bedouin women avoid direct assault (Al-Krenawi, 2000). Women have indirect ways of affecting these decisions by influencing their husbands or using their children to convey a message. In this context, female ways of resolving conflicts and influencing a husband's behavior can be characterized by the somatization of frustration; for example, by expressing jealousy in somatized forms or through indirect assaults, such as poisoning another wife's chickens. Another method of influence can be maintaining the status quo. For example, if the woman has young children and does not want to risk her husband divorcing her and taking away the children, she can avoid sexual contact with the husband or initiate more extreme avoidance, such as returning to her mother's house. More dramatically, she can stage an expression of her pain, such as a suicide attempt. Women can indirectly influence familial decisions through their children (Abu-Lughod, 1993; Holms, 2003). Outsiders assume that Arab women have no power because they lack legal rights. However, as shown above, Arab women are often strong and self-confident, especially in the rural communities where they work alongside their husbands and are economically productive. Thus, Bedouin women can influence decision making indirectly through their networks of kinship and friendship that have consequences for the men in their community (Tal, 1995; Yamini, 1996). Men may serve as heads of the family and are the speakers in the public sphere, but they consult privately with their wives before making decisions. The participation of women in the decision-making process is thus subtle and indirect, and so is their exercise of power (Afkhami, 1995; Cohen, 1999; Hijab, 1988; Yamini, 1996).

C. Use of Images Within Traditional Bedouin Culture

Visual art elements mostly consist of embroidery, weaving, and clay, elements that are used to decorate the women's area of the tent as well as people's clothes and camels' trappings (Fugel, 2002; Tal, 1995). A dominant art form of Islamic culture in general, including Bedouin culture, and indeed most nomadic cultures, is the male-dominated tradition of oral poetry and storytelling, which is used to convey collective history, values, and events that have taken place between the different nomadic tribes (Abu-Lughod, 1993; Al-Hammed, 2004; Bar Tzvi, 1986, 1999); calligraphy is also a male-dominated craft.

If we understand images and symbols to be a reflection of social and cultural values (Huss, 2010b; Mahon, 2000), then we can see these collective values expressed in traditional art forms. In the poetic calligraphy and fabric and clay crafts of the Bedouin, the aesthetic of abstract design stresses the importance of static balance, measure, and spacing. These designs challenge the eye with puzzles, and the repetitive patterns create a mystical sense of infinity (Irving, 1997; Kroup, 1995). Patterns are repeated, rotated, and varied in the context of harmony and order, all of the parts fitting into the whole. This reflects the values of traditional Bedouin culture, which views the individual as part of a complex, harmonious, and regulated whole (P. Allen, 1993; T. Allen, 1988; Fugel, 2002; Irving, 1997; Naasr, 2002). This aesthetic is in contrast to the role of art in Westernized culture, which, according to Western social values, embodies individuality, originality, and different or "authentic" experiences, often as a critique of the existing societal order. Indeed, even today, Kroup (1995) has found more decorative elements in Bedouin children's drawings than in more Westernized Jewish children's drawings in Israel.

Within traditional and gender-segregated cultures the masculine art forms of poetry and calligraphy use *words* to express the male experience. However, feminine art, often in craft forms, uses images to express cultural values and domestic power. For example, the traditional Bedouin embroidered dress represents an indirect expression of power. Embroidery has distinct patterns that signify information about marital status, number of children, and life transitions such as mourning. The dress also serves as a protective amulet; the bright colors embroidered over the breast area are used to protect milk production for children as well as to focus the male gaze. The bright colors can also be seen from afar in the desert, and thereby provide a protective element. Another type of fabric created by the women is the traditional Bedouin carpet, the *hadg*, which they weave. It is at the center of the tent, and all domestic interactions occur around it, symbolizing women's power in the domestic sphere. Traditional female crafts, such as embroidery, create an arena of social networks of help and competition as to the quality of the product (Fugel, 1992; Tal, 1980). This type of activity also serves as a source of surreptitious leisure in group gatherings, especially because many Muslim religious authorities view embroidering as an unnecessary source of pleasure. Additionally, specific embroidery patterns provide a collective identity that identifies a group from other groups. For example, Bedouin embroidery has different designs from those found in Palestinian embroidery (Tal, 1980).

As noted above, the traditional use of words is to express male experience, as in oral poetry and calligraphy, and images are used by traditional women, which forms a basis for using images as a form of expression with the Bedouin women in this case study (Huss, 2010b).

D. Bedouin Culture in Transition

The Bedouin in Israel are undergoing an intense and rapid cultural transition in the context of extreme poverty and conflict with the dominant Israeli state. This cultural transition is also typical of other rural and indigenous groups throughout the world.

According to researchers Ben-David (1981) and Meir (1997), this transition is commonly divided into three stages:

1. The Nomadic Pastoral Stage (pre-1948).
2. The Sedentarization Stage (1949–1966): The Israeli state limited Bedouin movement, but members of the Bedouin community were not allowed to enter the Israeli work force.

3. The Modernization Stage (1960–present): The Bedouin are settled into townships and enter the workforce (Meir, 2005).

In 1950, 2 years after the State of Israel was founded, the Bedouin living in Israel were moved to sedentary areas in the Negev that were less agriculturally productive. This policy triggered the ongoing political friction regarding landownership and the right of the Bedouin to continue a nomadic lifestyle (Barakat, 1993). Under the influence of the dominant Israeli culture, Bedouin society is now undergoing a change from a collective to an individualistic culture and from a nomadic lifestyle to one fixed in permanent settlements. According to the Center for Research on the Bedouin at Ben-Gurion University, the 100,000 contemporary Bedouin living in the Negev, located in southern Israel, account for 18% of the region's population. Roughly half of the Bedouin population living in this region resides within the seven recognized settlements, while the remaining half lives in tents and temporary dwellings within unrecognized settlements spread throughout the Negev region (Ben-David, 1981; Meir, 1997, 2005; Porat, 2009).

This process has resulted in a dramatic change in the social organization of the Bedouin community. Women and children, who previously played a central role in agriculture and husbandry, are no longer able to participate in the economic support system. Similarly, the transition from nomadism has devalued the traditional role of elders. Additionally, the surrender of social responsibilities to state authorities, who invest limited resources and often lack cultural relevance to the community, has resulted in the decline of the collective family support system (Kapri, Roznik, & Budekat, 2002; Lewando Hundt, 1978; Perez, 2001; Tal, 1995). Further, the move to a sedentary lifestyle eliminated the traditional pastoral source of livelihood for many Bedouin. Meanwhile, no new sources of livelihood, such as industry based on vocational training, have been created in the townships, thus increasing the poverty level. As a result, unemployment and child benefit support from the state have become the central sources of income for the impoverished Bedouin in the townships (Meir, 2005; Porat, 2009).

Like many similar indigenous peoples, the Bedouin are trapped in both an external struggle with the dominant society and an internal struggle with demographic and cultural changes caused by the transition from a nomadic to a sedentary lifestyle. This social transition and struggle include the context of extreme poverty and political conflict with the Jewish-Israeli state that is the result of oppression created by the severe neglect of this sector's public needs. The political conflict is partially due to the political conflict over lands that mars the relationship between the Bedouin and the state (Meir, 2005).

In 1999, the Center for Research of Bedouin Society at Ben-Gurion University published the first statistical yearbook on the Bedouin. This publication finally terminated the "invisibility" that characterized Bedouin society within the dominant Jewish literature. Since this breakthrough publication in 1999, several conferences on the Bedouin have been held at Ben-Gurion University. The conferences discussed educational and political strategies for conceptualizing and bettering the situation of the Bedouin community. Aside from the gross neglect of the Bedouin community that was discussed, these conferences also raised awareness that the transition to a sedentary lifestyle had shifted the manner in which the Bedouin build their self-identity and, further, created attempts to guide the Bedouin in their move to gain political recognition and rights. Nevertheless, contemporary Bedouin define themselves as both an indigenous and a colonized people (Abu-Said & Champagne, 2005). By defining themselves as an indigenous people, Bedouins embrace both a worldview and a call for more culturally relevant education, increased welfare services, and better living conditions. For example, Abu-Kuidar (1994), in her work on young girls' dropout rates from school, states that the educational system within the Bedouin community perpetuates discrimination by creating mixed schools that girls and young women cannot attend because there are boys there (rather than same-sex schools like those that exist in Jewish religious sectors in Israel) . Likewise, Al-Krenawi (2000), in his extensive work on culturally incompatible psychiatric services in Israel, describes the large dropout rate of patients from culturally irrelevant psychiatric services.

At the same time, Israel itself is struggling for identity; the values within the Bedouin community are different from those of the state at large, but Israel is not entirely a Western culture in and of itself. Indeed, post-Zionist theory claims that Arab and Jewish cultures are actually much more similar than different. For example, Abu-Baker (2002) claims that both Arab and Jewish males prefer to focus on national problems than to face the demands of equality for the women within their own societies.

E. Bedouin Women Within the Cultural Transition

Within the context of the transitions and struggles of the Bedouin community, the well-being of a woman often depends on the well-being of her male relatives and their reactions to the social climate (M. Cohen, 1999; Cwikel, 2002; Meir, 1997; Tal, 1995). Due to the breakdown of traditional family roles, such as brothers taking care of widows and elders, impoverished Bedouin women often become the responsibility of the welfare services of the state of Israel (Al-Krenawi, 2000; Kapri et al., 2002). However, these services are severely underfunded and understaffed, resulting in yet another form of oppression due to cultural misunderstandings and impoverished services. For example, as mentioned above, the government refuses to implement sex-segregated education for girls and women that would enable them to attend school after the onset of puberty.

Perez (2001) portrays a moving account of the difficulties of transposing Western values of social work into Bedouin culture. She describes a woman who is unable to flee from her abusive husband because of the lack of appropriate welfare services. She eventually escapes to a relative on foot at night, falling back on the traditional support system of the extended family, a system that is often already strained. Due to the forces of modernization, women are no longer busy with agricultural work; instead they are all in the house together for many hours, intensifying the traditional mother-in-law/new bride conflict. Contemporary young wives want more individual rights, such as private houses, more time alone with their husbands, and more control over their households, demands that further exacerbate the mother-in-law/daughter-in-law relationship (Al-Ataana, 1993, 2002; Lewando-Hundt, 1976). Another classic area of conflict occurs when the husband marries another wife. Polygamy has risen due to modernization, as men desire a more educated wife or wish to enhance their declining sense of power. The rise in polygamy has led to an increase in the conflicts among wives of the same husband. A number of studies reveal that older women yearn for a return to traditional ways. Yet, despite the inequality Bedouin women experience, the same study emphasized that younger Bedouin women prefer modernization. Abu-Lughod (1991) describes how Muslim men in general often embrace modernism while projecting traditional roles onto the women. While men enjoy the freedoms of modernity, women remain constricted, serving as a symbol of spiritual and cultural "purity" or authenticity (Abu-Lughod, 1993, p. 10). However, while the men in contemporary Bedouin communities limit women's opportunities, modernization itself allows for more freedom of movement as well as access to doctors and running water, as long as the women are not very poor and are allowed by Bedouin men to utilize these resources (Al-Ataana, 1993; M. Cohen, 1999; Cwikel, 2002).

F. Shifts in Modes of Visual Self-Expression in the Context of the Cultural Transition for Marginalized Bedouin Women

Traditional Bedouin crafts are on the decline because of the rise of Islamic movements that disapprove of time spent on embroidery, because embroidered clothes are worn less by the younger generations and mainly because embroidery can now be machine-made (Tal, 1995). For example, dresses are now made with one less panel, due to the dwindling practice of embroidery (Fugel, 2002; Lindsfore-Tapper & Ingham, 1997). At the same time, Western-style art is not taught in Bedouin schools, so, although traditional crafts are on the decline, the young women have not been provided with an alternative form of visual expression.

This is not the case for middle-class women who have access to Western art education, as can be seen in Ben Zvi and Lerer's (2001) book of Palestinian women artists that depict the experience of the male gaze and of the Zionist rule. In their compilation, Arab women's identity is expressed, through Western art discourses, as being fragmented by political and sexual oppression into multiple identities.

However, since 2004, the Bedouin educational system has started including art within its school services. According to the art teacher at the Key Center for Visual Arts in the Negev, more Bedouin women are training to become art teachers, which is a popular vocation because it does not require a high matriculation mark. Thus, the place of Westernized fine art within the Bedouin community may now start to extend beyond the upper and middle class. Furthermore, through Western visual media such as television, exposure to Western aesthetics and Western art traditions has expanded into all homes: Poor Bedouin women with access to a TV watch Arab TV channels and are exposed to Arab and Western aesthetic forms and images of Islamic modern culture. Similarly, although the practice of embroidery is dwindling overall, new designs are being created which reflect this new influence; for example, the symbol of a heart, a Western representation of love.

G. Similarities of the Above to Impoverished, Culturally Transitioning, or Indigenous Women in Global Culture

The rapid cultural transition from a rural to a sedentary urban culture is experienced by many women within different cultural contexts as they migrate from the countryside to town. For example, Shohat (1995) describes a similar process for impoverished women within indigenous Native American tribes in the United States. For them, sedentary life has strengthened patriarchal power and marginalized poor women to the outskirts of their community, making them invisible within their own culture. In terms of cultural transition then, many impoverished women in the world experience cultural transitions due to globalized work markets. These impoverished immigrant women living within a Westernized society tend to have difficulty making themselves and their needs heard within the public realm, which is similar to what the Bedouin women are now experiencing. Bedouin women are often misrepresented, stereotyped, and controlled by their husbands, who, themselves, are under stress and oppression. So these women have to deal with dual sets of oppression both inside and outside their culture (Afkhami, 1995; Canclini, 1996; Runyan & Peterson, 2009). However, the premise of third-world feminisms—and of the present analysis—is that the specific context of different cultural, social, and financial interactions has to be understood so as to unravel the types of oppressions that women experience within a specific social reality (Mohanty, 2003).

2 Working with Images
The Method Used in the Case Study

This case study does not wish simply to look at what women express but rather to hold a complex, multifaceted view of this "experience portrayed through images." This analysis will take into account the women's specific social oppressions and context, the group's specific context and concerns, and the influence of the gaze of the Jewish and Bedouin middle-class art therapists and researcher. This complexity is present in most intercultural interactions within social research and practice but is often not analyzed in terms of its overlapping influences and interactions. Despite my experience in research and in art therapy, this project led me into unknown territory. It brought me up against the limitations of my knowledge, experience, and current social theory.

Assumptions based in humanistic art-based research and phenomenological art therapy practices were no longer sufficient to explain the complex interaction of power relations, contexts, and contents that arose. The inclusion of a Bedouin social worker/art therapist as a coleader helped but did not fully elucidate the process expressed by the Bedouin women who were participating in my study because the social worker was a middle-class, Western-trained art therapist and thus distant from the women in different ways. Similarly, critical and postcolonial theories clarified the context of the participants' lives; however, the use of these theories alone would have come at the cost of understanding people from different classes and cultures whose own experience of reality has evolved from a web of projections and abuses of power.

These assumptions led me into pioneering territory, looking for methods to give complexity to the situation experienced by these women. It forced me to ask how images serve as a method for self-expression in different social contexts. How does it interact with the women's hybrid reality? And what kinds of narratives does it enable? Thus, instead of replicating another empowerment model or anthropological model, this case study aims to demonstrate how all these levels exist simultaneously.

As Spivak (Spivak & Guha, 1988) writes:

> It seems to me that finding the subaltern is not so hard, but actually entering into a responsibility structure with the subaltern, with responses flowing in both ways, learning to listen without this quick fix frenzy of doing good with an implicit assumption of cultural supremacy which is legitimized by unexamined romanticism, that's the hard part. (p. 292)

Following is a breakdown of how these questions were answered within this specific case study methodology:

Preliminary Questions

The preliminary questions that I aimed to answer in this research project were:

1. How do impoverished Bedouin women use images, in terms of content and in terms of form?
2. How does the use of image making help a cultural "outsider" understand the experience of these Bedouin women?
3. What roles did these images fulfill for the women?
4. What does this teach us about using images and arts processes for disadvantaged women?

Field of Research

The field of research was a set of groups for Bedouin women, which were jointly run and organized by the Department of Welfare Services, nongovernmental organizations (NGOs), and private franchises. The overall goal of these organizations was to help create empowerment amongst Bedouin women in the Negev area in Israel. This multiple case study took place in three preexisting women's groups. I gained access to the groups by offering my expertise in art implementation; I worked with a Bedouin cogroup implementer who was a master's student of mine and prefers to remain anonymous. The groups usually worked in small tin huts, club rooms, or basements of houses, places that were out of public view. The welfare group also had a room outside the welfare building in which the group met. All areas were private and had tables; I supplied the arts and crafts materials. Because the women lived in Bedouin townships, rather than within the traditional seminomadic lifestyle, they had presumably undergone some level of interaction with Western Israeli culture.

Research Strategy

The research strategy aimed to access the concerns and "natural" meeting places of the women. The art sessions were conducted as part of preexisting Bedouin women's groups and were customized to meet each group's needs as defined by the women. This was in accordance with feminist theory that suggests that methodology should begin by examining what issues are at stake for women and then developing questions only from that standpoint (Saulnier, 1996; Smith, 2002; Wolf, 1992). The research strategy that was negotiated with the women included four meetings over the course of the project for an hour and a half each, within each of the three groups for a total of 18 art hours. Each group defined its goals differently; for example, one group wanted to use images to help sort out their problems, one group wanted to make crafts, and one group wanted both of these things. The limited duration of the three meetings in the three different groups enabled me to remain an "outsider" while still having enough time to develop an art process and time-bounded relationships with the participants. The women were familiar with different experts entering the group to provide enrichment programs, such as workshops or lectures, so this experience fit into the aim of the group. Each of the three groups consisted of 15 to 20 women, who were aged between 20 and 50 years. The impoverished Bedouin women's drawings described in the following pages were gathered within these three groups and thus constitute a multiple case study design (Denzin & Lincoln, 2000; Patton, 1987). Yin (1993) defines such an approach as one in which a few slightly differing case studies are chosen to develop a theory about an issue central to the study.

The groups were led by me and an Arabic-speaking social worker, who had learned art skills in a master's degree program; further, she had extensive social work experience in the field of Bedouin women's groups as part of her practicum (she prefers to remain anonymous, so her name will not be mentioned here). Additionally, the long-term leader of the group was present during the sessions.

The Drawing Stage: Women's Interactions with Art in a Personal Context

Each woman was provided materials with which to draw her own picture or to make something using craft materials such as oils, pastels, paint, clay, fabric and thread, and colored silks. After each woman created her image, the images were laid out on the floor, at each creator's feet. A group discussion was initiated in which the women could ask each other questions about one another's images and each woman explained what she had undertaken. The role of the group leader was to help with the observation, reflection, and clarification of the images, as in focus groups, rather than to reframe, confront, or interpret the images, as is accepted in therapy groups. This participant-observer stance is cited as an appropriate tool for an unexplored field of research because it aids in developing questions to understand how people make sense of their reality (Eisenhardt, 2002). These insights create more specific questions and further challenges as the research proceeds. However, as will be shown, the art itself initiated transformative, therapeutic, and empowerment processes. The Jewish Israeli woman group leader can be understood as symbolizing the dominant culture and dominant power structure.

Recorded and Transcribed Data Sources

The recorded and transcribed data sources that these groups rendered included videotaped observation of the women while making art, the women's photographed images, the videotaped explanation of the images by the women in the group setting, and the groups' reactions to the joint "exhibition" of the artwork. Written sources included the researcher's field diary, the women's written summaries, transcripts of the group meetings from audio recordings, and relevant information on the context of the case, which was used to understand the drawings within the context of the specific group's circumstances and concerns.

Reflective Sources

Reflective sources included: the research diary; regular supervisory and peer supervision meetings between the research implementers and between the researcher and an external supervisor in relation to the group leadership; and partially structured interviews with some women from each group to clarify and to validate conclusions reached while analyzing the case studies as well as to gain a summative perspective of the experience (Hubberman & Miles, 2002). Three elements were kept at the center of the data: analyzing process, image, and the meanings that the women gave to the image. These elements were analyzed using a social theory of the interlocking oppressions that the women experience as impoverished women within an indigenous culture in transition that is in political conflict with the dominant Israeli culture (Denzin & Lincoln, 2000). This also was related to the researcher's positioning in terms of her power privileges within the setting.

Analysis of the Images

The images were analyzed through the women's explanation of the images according to phenomenological theories. This theory relies on the women's understanding of their own artwork as a central analytical tool. Phenomenological interpretation analyzes artwork within the context of the artist's own comments and understandings, rather than through an external analytical model. This method tries to understand the inherent content, or essence, of an experience as understood by the people experiencing it, and within the context of his or her group or culture. It uses a narrative style to describe the essence of the experience (Betinsky, 1995; Moustakas, 1994).

Second Analysis of the Images

The second analysis of the images was undertaken by the researcher, according to an observation of both form content and in the context of the social theory previously described (Huss, 2007, 2008, 2009a, 2012). This analysis aimed to relocate the images into the social contexts in which they were created (Denzin & Lincoln, 2000). The gaze and interaction with the dominant culture was considered to be symbolically exemplified and embodied through the researcher and thus impacted the art activity. This becomes another social analytical prism (Huss, 2009a).

By integrating phenomenological and critical theories, the analysis conceives of the art as a discourse that is both subjective and culturally embedded, and thus transcends the discourse that created it (Mahon, 2000; Silverman, 2000).

Qualitative Research

Qualitative research can be validated by including triangulation of data, postanalysis interviews, case comparison, the incorporation of nontypical data, and constant theoretical cross-checking (Silverman, 2000). As previously stated, the women's own drawings and explanations serve as an inherent form of validation of meaning within this research orientation. Additionally, all the researchers' analyses were peer analyzed with the Bedouin social worker and also with an external research group that included Jewish and Bedouin researchers. Consultations with other female Bedouin informants, such as leaders of empowerment groups and researchers in the Bedouin community, were used for self-monitoring (Andsell & Pavlicevic, 2001; Malchiodi & Riley, 1996).

Ethical Considerations

Ethical considerations included the multiple positions of the researcher who could, as group leader, cause the group to comply with her instructions as someone with power. This was the reason for the brief interactive duration of the researcher within the group and for the inclusion of the full-time group leader. The interaction between the researcher, a Jewish woman, and the group participants, impoverished Bedouin women, is analogous to the typical situation these women face in their daily lives. Thus, while this interaction is indeed problematic, it provides a crucial opportunity to understand how women create their "speech acts" in relation to the dominant Israeli-Western culture that engulfs them. Ultimately, this interaction became a prism for analysis (van Kleef, De Dreu, & Manstead, 2004; Wolf, 1992).

The issues of interpretation, exhibition, record keeping, and ownership are ethical issues within any type of art interaction and are much debated within the art therapy literature (Andsell & Pavlicevic, 2001; Moon, 2000). For example, art and words can be seen as a commodity that is taken away from its creator or speaker and used for the gain of the researcher. In order to ensure both confidentiality and to clarify the research aims to participants, all research subjects signed an agreement to allow their work to be used within the context of the research. Their desire not to have the work displayed outside of the group did not hinder their opportunity to join the group in any way. Despite the presence of consent forms, it is important to note that due to the cultural norm of compliance with perceived authority and unfamiliarity with research, Bedouin women may feel pressure to give up a wish for privacy. All the pictures created were scanned into a computer and then returned to the women themselves. All the images are completely anonymous, and any information that may disclose the identity of the women through the use of their choice of words around the picture has been changed. When the participants expressed distress during the sessions, the group implementers referred women to individualized help as needed, creating a beneficial service for the women. Additionally, the group did not employ a "one off" method of entering and taking away their drawings, but rather, met with the women over the course of four meetings, which was enough time to process the meaning of the art for the women and to deal with disturbing contents (Malchiody & Riley, 1996).

Overall, the above method will be further discussed and woven into the fabric of this book as a whole. Questions that are raised from this and that are part of working with images in social research and practice include the following issues:

1. How is art or image making defined, and who defines it? In this case, an effort was made to define image making with the women in the workshops.
2. What are the power relations between the participants and the implementer of the image making, and how does this impact the images created? In this research, the differences in power between researcher and participants (middle-class Jewish and Bedouin women and impoverished Bedouin women) became an analytical prism in and of itself.
3. Who has the power to define and to analyze images, and what analytical prisms are used within this definition? This research moved

beyond content, as in arts-based research, and phenomenology, as in art therapy, and included a specifically contextualized social prism as an additional way to understand images.
4. What constitutes a therapeutic use versus research use of images? In this research project, the role of the group leader was not to intervene, as is expected in an art therapy group so as to confront and to transform meaning, but rather to enable the observation, reflection, and clarification of the pictures (Betinksy, 1995).
5. Who owns the images? These questions are relevant to research, therapy, empowerment, or social action projects that use images. They point to the fact that the use of images does not bridge or circumvent issues of power but rather are an additional medium in which they are concretized.

Altogether, these areas of concern and methodological and theoretical challenges aim to explore how I, as a representative of the dominant culture, position myself and restrain my preconceptions in order to actively "see" the images of the marginalized Bedouin women within the context of their social reality.

3 Bedouin Women's Images on the Level of Content

The Bedouin women's images will be analyzed or explained first by the women who drew them and second by the researcher, based in the social context of the Bedouin as a community in cultural transition and sedantarization, from the position of poverty, as described in the former chapter.

A. Outside Spaces and Mobility

Women's Explanations of the Images

One of the most dominant wishes expressed by the group participants was the ability to be mobile, to be able to get out of the house.

> What we most need? We need to go on a holiday, to get out of here, to have a change of scenery because we can't travel or go visiting without men. We are stuck at home. The welfare offices took us for two days to a hotel with our children. It was heaven.

Although the sea is only 45 minutes away from the township, many of the women stated that they had never been there. The following woman drew her wish to go to the sea. She explained (see Figure 1, Image 2): "I wish to go to the sea, I have been to the sea and I love the sea. I wish to go more to the sea. I want to learn lots of things, also to drive, and then I can also go to the sea." This motive was continued in the next picture, where one woman explained her wish to take the children to swim in the pool (see Figure 1, Image 2).

> I'm just drawing my dreams, to go to a pool. I want to go to a pool like this and to have all the children swim in the pool. Now I want to dive into that pool. I went there once but I cannot take my children to such a pool because I can't drive.

Another woman described pleasure in being in a traditional type of outside space. "I remember as a child, going out with the sheep, I loved going out with the sheep" (see Figure 1, Image 1). A hindrance to mobility is the difficulty in obtaining a driver's license and in acquiring access to a car. In the following image the woman explained: The artist had written the words "a journey of peace and not war" above the picture. She described how she has, after many failures, completed her theory driving test, but must now find the money to learn to drive before the theory test expires, as had happened to her before. The woman said how important her driver's license was for her, as it would enable her to be mobile. She drew a stop sign in the drawing because there are so many automobile accidents within the Bedouin villages and townships (see Figure 1, Image 4).

The following example is part of the group discussion around the obvious differences between inside and outside, and about the preference for outside:

Participant 2:   "I see your outside area is much richer than inside; you also prefer to be outside?"
Participant 1:   "Yes, outside is important for children."
P 2:   "Why? What does outside give to children?"
P 1:   "A different world, freedom, movement, independence."
P 2:   "Sand, the feeling of sand."
P 1:   "The air, the wind, the smell of the wind."

This richness of outside versus inside is demonstrated in the women's images of inside and outside.

Social Analysis of Images

We have seen that the women yearn for mobility; traditionally, Bedouin women had mobility within the overall area of the tribe and occasionally made trips to different tribes to visit relatives (Meir, 2005; Tal, 1995). However, different elements within townships serve to inhibit poor Bedouin women's mobility. From this social perspective, the women's pictures can be understood as a wish to enter Western culture, which enables mobility, or a return to traditional culture, which also enables a different type of mobility. For example, one of the women drew an Israeli-style "beach" in which people were physically present and showering; the image was a metaphor which included a Western type of nature, compared to the image of the sheep, which depicted the traditional culture in nature. (see Figure 1, Image 1)

The second image of the pool is another Western allusion, a man-made body of water, rather than a water source in the desert. Swimming pools are built in all the Jewish settlements in the area, but not in the Arab settlements, due to both cultural and financial considerations. However, despite its physicality as a real space, a swimming pool is described by the women as a dream; indeed, due to the interacting levels of poverty, gender, and culture, swimming in a pool is a dream for these women; thus, one woman says that she wishes to jump into the pool now, but also that she is "only drawing her dreams."

In the picture of the sheep and the tent, the woman describes traditional spaces. As previously stated, the Bedouin self-define themselves as an indigenous people (Abu-Said & Champagne, 2005). Nomadism implies a different relationship between inside and outside spaces and between private and public spaces than is found in sedentary communities (Mernissi, 2003; Tuhiwai-Smith, 1999). For example, a tent creates an intrinsic relationship between inside and outside spaces as compared to a house, which is more closed to the outside. Indigenous theories define the inherent connection between inside and outside or with nature as something to be reincorporated into the indigenous knowledge base that is being lost (Abu-Said & Champagne, 2005); this connection with nature is also apparent in the image of outside versus inside.

The limitation on mobility that the women currently experience is, as stated, the result of the meeting point between enforced sedentarization, impoverished state resources, and cultural limitations initiated by the Bedouin patriarchy. According to Tal (1995), the possibility of work and free movement outside the tribe is perceived by Bedouin men as a threat to the traditional roles of women. As a result, women are increasingly under men's control and increasingly limited to the house. Traditional spaces are also no longer available and can only be remembered. Mobility is thus constricted from different sources: First, as a result of poverty, the women cannot afford a car to be mobile. Second, in the context of a lack of state resources, the bus services are inadequate in the Bedouin townships and unrecognized settlements. Third, in the context of cultural gendered norms, a Bedouin traditional woman cannot travel publicly unless she is accompanied by a man. These different types of constrictions or oppressions—lack of state resources along with cultural and financial constrictions—collude to inhibit women's mobility (Al-Ataana, 2002; Cwikel, 20021; Mernissi, 2003; Mohanty, 2003; Perez, 2003). The different types of limitations interlock to leave the women without either traditional or Western spaces and mobility. This lack of mobility is in contrast to middle-class Bedouin women, who can access mobility by driving a private car.

B. Inside Spaces: Houses

Poverty makes achieving a home nearly impossible for poor Bedouin women not protected by men. As previously stated, the first problem is the lack of money to afford a house:

Houses are most important for us. I have my house; it has broken windows, a few mattresses on the floor, one room. We don't have enough blankets. Last night we couldn't sleep, all of us, we were so cold and the wind blew through the broken window. But it's my hut and it gives me safety. I'm glad I have it. My dream is to fix it, to plant flowers, to make it nice, to give each child his space (see Figure 1, Image 7).

Bedouin Group Leader (GL): "What did you draw?"
Group Participant (P 1): "I drew a house; I want a house. These are the rooms."
GL: "What is most important about your house?"
P 1: "Strong walls—and also I want to plant flowers in my own garden."
P 2: "I am interested in your picture; I also want a house, alone. I live with my five children with my parents. I'm divorced and I want a house alone." (See Figure 1, Images 6 and 7.)

"Now I have a small house, but it's better than before, although it's small. I'm happy to be in it—it is full of colors. Before my divorce my husband was violent and I had a black house."

However, houses can also be a form of confinement, as described below (See to Figure 1, Images 7 and 8):

P 1: [Crying] "I have a big house but I am lost, I am lonely in it. I sit and watch TV all day. I am in front of the TV all day in my house, I feel like an ant."

Social Analyses

Within the context of poverty and cultural constraint, a house is very difficult to acquire due both to a lack of income and to a lack of independence for women. The house symbolizes space, independence, and physical and emotional security. However, a house, while desired, is also confining, in terms of cultural norms that can restrict women indoors, leaving them bored and alone. If we compare this to the literature describing the typical descriptions of the house as the bustling women's area and as a center of activity, then the above descriptions are parallel to the Arab feminist literature describing the modern, Westernized house as limiting for Arab women (Abu-Lughod 1993; Lewando-Hundt, 1978; Mernissi, 2003; Ong, 2003; Sabbagh, 1997). Abu-Lughod (1993) claims that, traditionally, the women's community was an independent sphere that included gossip, sexual language, rituals, and hosting guests, whereas modernization combined with Islam "wants to place women firmly in their homes under their husbands' control" (p. 19). Simultaneously, due to the limitations on hunting and the nomadic lifestyle, men have taken over roles that were previously under women's control (Tal, 1995). This collusion of social limitations makes inside as well as outside spaces, and, most importantly, the ability to transition freely between inside and outside, impossible for these women. This inhibits the women's ability to reach additional spaces such as education, social venues, and more complex self-actualization on all of Maslow's levels (Maslow, 1970). Because these oppressions emerge from different sources, it is confusing for the women to know what to wish for. As previously stated, compared to this predicament, middle-class Bedouin women do have access to mobility and to houses. Although the literature described their dilemmas and the complex cultural splits that they experience, the middle-class women have the resources to undertake the negotiations between traditional and Western spaces (Abu-Kuidar, 1994; Levi-Wiener, 2004). This situates poverty interacting with gender as the most pervasive of oppressions (Mohanty, 2003; Moor, 1997).

C. Wish for Education (see Figure 2, Image 1)

As a young woman I dreamed of becoming a teacher, but because I had young brothers and sisters to take care of, formal study remains only a dream. Now I have my own children and it is still a dream.

Yes, I agree; going to school as a child was the happiest time of my life. I wish to "climb back up the path to studies" (see Figure 2, Image 2).

Social Analyses

Figure 1, Images 9 and 10 show the experience of poverty, as well as the failure to find a way of transcending poverty. The Bedouin as a population transitioning from nomadic to modern status is one of the poorest segments of Israeli society. Currently, 70% of the Bedouin live below the poverty line. According to the *Statistical Year Book of the Negev Bedouin* (1986), at least 20% of the men and 90% of the women are unemployed. The community suffers from heavy drug abuse; there is a 70% drop-out rate from high school. Among women, 90% do not complete their high school education. When men are oppressed, women are doubly oppressed: The negative outcome of societal changes on the female population specifically is shown in statistical studies of Bedouin women's health. A study conducted by Cwikel (2002) points to increased male violence, intense interconnected poverty, social problems, and health problems such as depression, anemia, and difficulty in accessing health care (Cwikel, 2002; Tal, 1995). One way to overcome poverty is to work; however, Bedouin women are not always allowed to work outside the house with strangers. Another method is to pursue an education to become a professional worker; however, again, cultural as well as financial elements collude to prevent an education, which is a central strategy for transcending poverty.

D. Shifting Spaces Between Children and Adults

One woman described her struggle to raise children in poverty

> I am like a tree, trying to be strong. How can I be a mother to children when I can't give them the things they need? I am trying to let the children ask for things, to give them what they need. My biggest problem is lack of money.

The following woman describes experiencing the children as emotionally lost to her (see Figure 2, Image 4):

> I have ten children but I am lonely. This is my heart, I drew my heart. My heart is the only thing I have left … I drew my child as a flower, he is my flower, but he has gone to drugs, I am so unhappy.

Another issue is the lack of a father figure, or of negotiating relationships with polygamous fathers:

P 1: [Made a small clay statue of a mother and child that she took with her] "This is the main joy of the women—to have children."
P 2: "But when they are older, it is hard. For instance, I have problems with my daughter, who wants to be with her father and to leave me alone."
P 1: "This is true."
P 3: "You should let your daughter go with her father, because for her it is important to think of her father."
P 2: "But she leaves me all alone. She goes with his new wife and his children, and I am left all alone."
P 3: "Still, you must think of her. You can visit a friend."

A widow described the problems of not having a protective father figure for her children: "I am a widow. I have problems with my children now, as my husband's brother hit the children. I don't go to sleep every night until the brother and children are asleep. I am tired. My house was taken away from me." As a widow, she could not continue living alone with her children.

Social Analyses

To summarize the above examples, the women in this study repeatedly described their children as "lost" to them; in other words, too far away, due to cultural transition, poverty, lack of status of the mother, and lack of the authority of a father figure, where the father is absent due to unemployment and his declining status, or due to polygamy where the father is more interested in his latest wife and children (M. Cohen, 1999). The children are described as "lost" to their mothers, not due to lack of love or to the women's lack of skills, but rather due to the interaction of poverty, lack of status, and the loss of traditional child raising ways.

It is important to understand how the cultural transition redefined the role of children and thus educational values: Women and children previously played a central role in agriculture and husbandry, but are now no longer able to participate in the economic support system. Older women who could not work in agriculture and who were once respected as having the traditional role of elders, are now also devalued. Overall, the externalization of social responsibilities to state authorities, who invest limited resources and often lack cultural relevance to the community, has resulted in the decline of collective family support and funds that can help to educate children as part of a collective tribe with interactive roles (Cwikel, 2002; Kapri, Roznik, & Budekat, 2002; Perez, 2001).

For example, if children and parents interact in a collective or tribal space, then, as Jayanthi (2002) writes, children learn by being near adults and observing adult behavior. However, living alone in a small house does not enable the children to learn from the mother and her interactions with the other women in the tribe. Simultaneously, due to the limitations on hunting and nomadic lifestyle, men have taken over roles that were previously under women's control in the home, such as overseeing children's education.

In addition to state and welfare power over the women, Western values are also taught to the women and influence their way of bringing up children. For example, many daycare centers have been opened so that women can enter the workforce (see Figure 2, Image 5).

"Here are all the things a baby needs: a bottle, a diaper, a cot." In the image above, Westernized influences in childcare are expressed, as the woman defines what a child needs according to a list of Western commodities. We see that these items float in space, as if disconnected to the inherent structure of how women bring up children. A list of metonymic elements are placed randomly on the page, rather than organized into a coherent spatial relationship. The elements "float" in space, as if out of context to the women's real lives: things wished for and imagined, but not integrated into their reality. This is in comparison to the pictures of landscapes that are coherent and rich in terms of composition and color (Huss, 2004). Sullivan (2001) describes the move to modernism in Arab states as disempowering women through a wide range of reeducation tactics. However, since the impoverished women in this study cannot, as shown above, afford to fully undergo the processes of modernization, they become powerless in the eyes of their children. This image of powerlessness is reflected back to them, although they fight to protect, fix, and provide for their children, as shown in the narratives. Abu-Kuidar (1994) describes how the state does not enable gender-segregated schools; so girls often leave school at puberty and forfeit an education. Overall, the Bedouin educational system is severely impoverished. Thus, poor children, like women, do not have access to Westernization or even to traditional educational values. The shifting roles of women and children disempowers the relationship between them, creating such distance that the children are "lost" and not seen by the mothers or alternatively that the women feel they have lost control and influence within their children's lives (Meir, 1997). This is due to the shifting roles within the community as a whole and to the shifting roles of Bedouin women in relation to Bedouin men.

E. Shifting Spaces between Bedouin Women and Men

One woman described women's need for men's protection through the metaphor of a tree (see Figure 2, Image 6): This lack of protection is equated with the lack of water for the tree and is described in the following image as:

Another theme was the demand for the right to enter processes of Westernization for women as well as for men; for example, one woman demanded the right to dress in Western-style clothing as the men do (see Figure 2, Image 8). In the following image, the woman described how she indirectly resists her husband's power (see Figure 2, Images 9 and 10).

Social Analyses

Traditionally, men are given the power as well as the responsibility for ensuring the well-being of women. Indeed, Bedouin values assign the responsibility for protecting women to their male relatives; however, the rise in poverty and individualistic social organization among the Bedouin has resulted in the extended family's inability to protect women or to accompany them when they want to move outside their settlement (Meir, 1997; Tal, 1995). Thus, on the one hand Bedouin men can provide familial protection to women, and, on the other, they can inhibit their freedom; for example, the participant who compared women to being plants and men to being their gardeners describes women as passive objects and men as the "cosmos" that sends down rain. Yet, the image also places an indirect responsibility or demand on the men: They must care for the women. This woman uses a proverb to indirectly state that if men continue to "water" or protect women, then women can blossom.

Conversely, the last two women demanded more freedom, or the right to become Western, as men do. Impoverished Bedouin women are often constricted as a result of the unequal changes in Bedouin culture between men and women. Abu-Lughod (1991) describes how Muslim men often embrace modernism while continuing to project traditional roles onto the women. Thus, while men enjoy the freedoms of modernity, women remain constricted, serving as a symbol of spiritual and cultural "purity" or authenticity. The woman above, however, demands the right to "dress up and be pretty," defining the path to modernity through the symbolic meaning of clothes. We see that paradoxically, by demanding the right to dress in a Western fashion, women resist Bedouin men, in order to attract them, which then repositions men as dominant. Abu-Lughod (1993) interprets the demand to express sexuality as a form of rebellion. She writes,

> Even today, young Bedouin women in Egypt try to resist their elders and the kin-based forms of domination they represent by embracing aspects of a commoditized sexuality—buying makeup and negligees that carry with them both new forms of control and new freedoms. (p. 13)

The demand to dress in a Western style symbolizes the only form of entry into the process of Westernization that is open to poor women. Middle-class Arab feminists define the issues that concern Arab women as education and voting, rather than as sexual self-expression (Sabbagh, 1997). However, impoverished women, who do not have access to education or to social and financial power, express their resistance through visual codes of dress. This is similar to the use of the Bedouin-embroidered dress, cited in the literature survey as a way to communicate power, such as status and number of children. It is the way that women display power to other women (Lindsfore-Tapper & Ingham, 1997).

The women state that a woman "has hands" but is not allowed to use them. When the men in the family are oppressed, the women are doubly oppressed. As stated before, poor Bedouin men who are unemployed and do not have the traditional activities of agriculture and hunting have taken over roles that were previously under women's control in the home, such as overseeing the education of the children. Overall, the women ask for traditional protection as well as the right to enter modernity. At present, because women lack financial resources, they have neither types of support from men, which leaves them with the experience of being a "black cloud not connected to anything" (Figure 1, Image 9).

On the other hand, the women have indirect ways of resisting the power of men; for example, in Figure 2, Image 10, where the woman says "yes, yes" but does not do what her husband says. The woman shows how she indirectly resists the men who are not at home within her traditional space and area to exercise power. This example illustrates tactics of indirect resistance used by third-world women (Ong, 2003; Shohat, 1995).

Interestingly, apart from this doll, there are no other images that are drawn of men as compared to women. We receive an abstract "Godly" impression of men, while women are drawn and compared to plants, such as palm trees, giving them a "grounded" level. Mernissi (2003) describes men as obeying God and women as obeying men. The difficulty in locating or describing men's power is similar to descriptions of patriarchal power as an unbound force that is not limited to a single institution and is, thus, difficult to fight against. The women's struggles show how feminist struggles must be defined within specific contexts and cultures, rather than as universal elements (Mohanty, 2003; Taylor, Gilligan, & Sullivan, 1995).

F. Relationship to Jewish State

Another power holder is the Israeli state. One woman described her interaction with the state as a struggle to receive a permit for building; she lives in one of the unrecognized villages (Figure 2, Image 11):

> I am in a house with no permit. I am like on an upward hill trying to get back my house (cries). This is a hill. I have no building permit; I feel I am on a steep hill, going up, and never reaching the top. I build my house, they break it. I am always climbing up (cries).

Conversely, another woman describes how she is protected from her violent husband by the state: "My husband has an emotional problem; it can't be fixed. He would hit me and the children. Now it's okay because if he hits me or the children, he's immediately back in jail."

Another women described wanting to look like a Western Israeli rather than a Bedouin woman (Figure 2, Image 13). Another woman drew a modern, secular Israeli woman and a traditional Bedouin woman holding hands. She explained: "The traditional women is trying to pull the modern women in her direction, but she doesn't want to go ..." (see Figure 2, Image 14).

Social Analyses

We have seen that the state can both oppress the women by not giving them access to housing or travel, and it can also protect them against violent husbands. This social oppression interacts with other types of oppressions, such as the status of women in the Bedouin culture. Thus, different power holders collude from different directions. The Bedouin women are simultaneously controlled both by the state and by the Bedouin patriarchy, creating a complicated and often oppositional relationship between power holders.

On a more direct level, the Bedouin woman is connected to health and welfare services, where she interacts with many Jewish female social workers, health care workers, and others who are mainly female (Perez, 2001). We see relationships of emulation, competition, and conflict with these power holders. For example, in the picture of a thin, blond woman, who is so thin and pale that she nearly disappears into the page, it is as if the woman is "rubbing out" her real image as a large middle-aged Bedouin woman in traditional dress. On the other hand, peer analyses of the images by Bedouin women pointed out that the blonde woman can also be seen as a reference to Russian immigrant women in the area who often become mistresses of Bedouin men, taking them away from their wives; in this specific context, the picture gains additional meanings (see Figure 2, Image 13).

G. Summary of Social Analyses of Images on the Level of Content

The above images show how the physical and emotional spaces of Bedouin women, in relation to others, have shifted. Thinking in terms of space rather than abstract concepts helps to reveal the interaction of different types of oppression that creates the lack of space or inability to enter Western processes or to maintain traditional culture. For example, the wish to go to the sea was seen as being impossible to achieve due to lack of money; but the inability to go to the sea is also due to the lack of the dominant culture's travel infrastructure and the lack of the traditional culture's sanction for a women to travel alone. Poor Bedouin women cannot afford private cars and are not permitted to travel alone by bus. From the position of poverty, the women in this study do not have the resources to negotiate for houses, mobility, traditional or Western culture, or relationships with Muslim men, Jewish state representatives, or their own children. Overall, the set of images describes a social context that follows the literature on the multiple levels of oppression that the women face: Compared to this, literature on middle-class Bedouin women describes how they utilize the cultural transitions and shifts so as to gain access to education, mobility, and houses (see Figure 2, Image 1).

The drawing and its explanation help to make concrete the exact qualities the woman defines as important, for example, in a house (i.e., space and freedom, emotional warmth). However, the limitations of mobility make these same qualities of a house confining. It is as if she has had a chance to walk into the drawn house and has realized what it is like to be inside. The solution offered by the woman to this potential isolation is to leave the house and to travel, or to go outside. However, the women also lack mobility. This leaves them with no spaces, inside or outside, that are satisfying.

The images reveal this lack of space, and the emotional pain and confusion that this creates. The use of images enables both the women themselves and outside observers to experience how the dynamics of these interlocking levels of oppression work simultaneously within a single image. Spivak (1993), whose work has focused on revealing the marginalized voice of Indian women, poignantly expresses the multiple levels of oppression these women experience in the following quote:

> [They are] shuttled between different levels of oppression ... disappearing not into a pristine nothingness, but into a violent shuttling which is the displaced figuration of the third world women, caught between tradition and modernization. (p. 292)

The social analysis of the images that focuses on specific situations reveals this experience of "violent shuttling." The images become, in Abu-Lughod's terms (1991), "ethnographies of the particular...that capture the cultural and social 'forces' that are only embodied in the actions of individuals in time and space" (p. 156).

A social reading of the images impacts the description of the most basic metonyms of the women's lives as extending from the physical to the emotional and reveals how these intersecting oppressions permeate every experience, making the personal political, even if it is not defined as such by the women themselves. This is at the base of a social reading of images.

However, a compositional reading of these images will render levels of experience that show how the women experience and react to their reality. The women experience intense pain and helplessness, but also constantly work to redefine and to indirectly resist the intersection of oppressions and poverty. The next chapter will demonstrate this by shifting focus onto the compositional elements of the images, which include the process of construction, aesthetic mechanisms, and types of interpretation and impact upon others.

4 Pain and Resilience as Seen in the Compositional Elements of the Bedouin Women's Images

A. Mapping Experience Into Space

As shown in the previous chapter, the impoverished Bedouin women's images make apparent the lack of spaces that they experience due to their multiple levels of oppression. An image at its most elementary level organizes contents into the spatial area of the page, revealing this lack of spaces. This organization defines the relative size and physical distance between objects in terms of subject, background, and interaction between elements that create the narrative or content of the image (Huss, 2012). Examples from the previous chapter that include spatial organization include the distance from the places dreamed of by the women, such as nature and trips, the confinement of people into houses, and the size and organization of houses, as well as the relative size, distance, metaphors, symbols, and compositional contrasts used to describe the distance of the Bedouin women from children, men, and non-Bedouin women. Once a space is "mapped out," its limitations in the context of the interlocking types of oppression previously described are revealed. For example, we saw before that once the "dream house" was drawn or mapped out, some women then described it as isolating and boring.

The women also used the page to portray their isolation and loneliness in terms of being alone, or in terms of unanswered requests for help or freedom from others, such as Jewish women, Bedouin men, and the state. For example, the women who believe that their children are emotionally "lost" to them do not even draw their children on the page, the distance from other women, and the woman alone in her house. The picture of the black cloud and the picture of the very thin blonde woman, for example, display a lack of contour, or, in other words, a lack of defined space within the drawn body; a lack of space for the self (see Figure 2, Images 13 and 7).

To elaborate, the woman who experiences herself as a "black cloud" because there is no man in her life represents herself with no contours. Conversely, the woman who wants to be thin and blonde creates an image made up only of lines, with no space between the lines. In other words, the compositional elements such as spatial divisions and contours depict the woman's emotional experience of the social content. Colors, as well as the shapes and relative size of objects on the page convey emotional meaning. For example, in Figure 1, Image 6, we see a black house used to describe a house when the abusing husband lived there. Similarly, a black cloud or very pale women was defined in terms of colors.

The women wished for Western spaces, depicted in the spatial relationships on the page as wishes for mobility, freedom, and "space for each child." Because the empty page is a symbolic as well as a concrete space, the spaces between objects on the page and the way the objects were rendered become symbolic depictions of this wish for Western culture. The spatial organization of the images *shows*, rather than *tells*, how impoverished women are left with no space and with no agency to be either sedentary or mobile, traditional or Western; they have no spaces within which to build defined but connected relationships with men, children, or each other (Mills, 1991, 1997; Spivak, 1987).

B. Resistance to Lack of Spaces

By being revealed, the above described lack of space actually becomes a site for resistance and a means to find solutions. One could define the representation of lack of space as taking up symbolic space on the page or as symbolically reclaiming space. The woman who drew a large and detailed house (Figure 1, Image 7) symbolically reclaimed space.

C. Metonyms and Wishes

In addition to use and division of space, the symbolic language chosen to define the content becomes a symbolic depiction of reality: Many women used the form of a wish to draw things that they do not have, from concrete things such as houses, to abstract things such as education, and emotional things such as male protection. The images of the concretized wishes, by definition, contain the opposing reality that describes what the women lack: houses, education, Western clothing, cars, and the beach. All these images were drawn as metonyms that also become symbols of wealth and Western values.

Wishes are a compatible form for traditional culture in that they show what is lacking but do not directly demand what is lacking. Images do not create direct conflict with power holders, such as Bedouin men or the Jewish state. The solutions to these lacks can be derived from a religious faith that God will provide (Afkhami, 1995; Naasr, 2002). Wishes are thus a culturally compatible symbolic form. The concrete as well as the emotional and compositional contents of wishes drawn onto a page

40   *Art as a Speech Act from the Margins*

and made visible indirectly create a confrontation with the lack of these things wished for.

As shown in the former chapter, on the level of a hybrid cultural reality, for the Bedouin women living a life between two discourses makes even wishing for things difficult. A large Western house will still be lonely without other women, as in traditional culture; further, such a house will be lonely and restrictive without the cultural sanction to leave it. Likewise, Western baby paraphernalia floats without context in the woman's drawing (see Figure 2, Image 5), as a nontraditional element; thus it becomes difficult even to define what to wish for, just as the same wished-for house in reality can be an experience of loneliness and confinement. This together creates much pain that is also conveyed symbolically through the women's drawings.

D. Symbols of Pain

As previously stated, the interlocking levels of oppression and, most intensely, of poverty, create much pain, which is described in the following example (see Figure 3, Image 3):

> We are like birds looking for food. I want to eat bread with shawarma, but I don't have money. I can't, so I don't. I eat pita alone, and that's OK, I feel better when I control my spending. I need help to understand how much money I have.

Symbols that are drawn, such as birds, contain more levels of meaning than metonymic or illustrative drawings. They include both cognitive and emotional content that cannot be encompassed within a single word (Furth, 1998; Jung, 1974; Riley, 1997; Save & Nuutinen, 2003).

The Bedouin women's images show how the distance from a wish, as well as the confusion over what to wish for, is a meeting with pain; the broader frame of symbols or metaphors becomes a way to express this pain. Within Islamic and Bedouin culture, symbols of nature and animals are culturally accepted forms for expressing emotion (Abu-Lughod, 1988; Al-Hamamdeh, 2004; Allen, 1998). Over the course of this project, we saw images of ants, cows, horses, trees, and flowers being used symbolically in the women's artwork. We saw symbols of ants, cows, horses, fish, trees, and flowers in the women's images.

> "I did a picture of a fish in the sea. The fish is alone, because I feel alone."

> "I am lonely as an ant, sitting and watching TV all day at home" (see Figure 3, Image 4).

> "I am standing, thank God, and I am like the tree because I am trying to be strong and connected to the ground although my branches feel the wind."

In the example of the woman as a tree struggling in the wind, the visual gestalt shows the intense emotional flooding of the tree as it is pushed around by the wind that is also a way of representing types of oppression or fate. At the same time, the verbal elaboration around the image reveals the woman's strength in her efforts to "stay connected to the ground."

E. Embodied Symbols

In the next example the tree loses its projective distance in nature and becomes personified: the tree is crying (see Figure 3, Image 5).

> My son had a car accident, and since then he has changed. I've sought help everywhere, but no one has helped me; all day I cry because my child is lost. I gave birth to him [crying]. I drew me as a crying tree.

The next example shifts even further away from nature, and portrays a body part as a symbol (see Figure 3, Image 6). In the spiral, the symbolism has moved into the body, specifically, the mind. The woman's mind is working and turning, but again, due to her circumstances, she cannot find a solution; further, the mind has no way of expressing its confusion outwardly other than spiraling in on itself.

In the following picture, the symbolism has moved from the mind to the heart (emotions). This image utilizes a Western symbol of the heart as love (see Figure 3, Image 7).

> I am divorced. I got married at 15 and I have ten children. The marriage started okay, and then after two years the problems started when my brother died. My husband has an emotional problem; it can't be fixed. He would hit me and the children. Now it's okay. Now I am okay, I just want someone to listen to me. I have ten children but I am lonely. This is my heart; I drew my heart. My heart is the only thing I have left.

This use of body parts is similar to the process of somatization of pain in the body that is characteristic of women (Huss & Cwikel, 2008a; Karaz, 2005). However, here the pain is projected into a symbol and distanced onto the page rather than being swallowed into the body. The meeting between emotion and cognition when observing and explaining the drawn symbol enables the woman to define the pain within a specific reality as socially constructed from the outside, rather than as an inherent illness inside her.

F. Traditional versus Western Symbols

As previously stated, nature is an accepted metaphor for intense emotion that is expressed indirectly and decoratively. However, we see above that there is a gradual shift from nature to body parts: Similarly, even the trees, despite the use of a traditional art form, are single and alone on the page, rather than being depicted in a group of trees in a patterned configuration of nature symbolizing a harmonious whole that represents collective values as in the following figure (see Figure 3, Image 8).

In Figure 3, Image 4, the woman who drew the tree is using a traditional symbol for emotion but is appropriating it to express her isolated reality. This is a new interpretation of a traditional symbol. The use of wishes, metonyms, and symbols from nature was defined above as traditional aesthetic mechanisms of Bedouin culture. However, the symbols utilize traditional symbolic contents in new compositional forms, such as a single tree rather than a patterned configuration of an infinite number of trees. This usage expresses the shift to individualism from collectivist cultures and portrays the experience of isolation of impoverished women within the experience of cultural transition. Thus, the aesthetic forms of a culture, as previously seen, are always dynamic and changing in order to incorporate new experience. This illustrates how people constantly reinterpret culture and also use cultural symbols to reinterpret their experience (Furth, 1998; Jung, 1974). However, impoverished women in a process of cultural transition do not always have a symbolic language with which to redefine experience. For example, in the case of the Bedouin women in the present study, due to the dwindling of traditional crafts and lack of Western art education, both are areas that are no longer available to the women as an outlet for their feelings and as a space to partake in the redefinition of cultural narratives (see Chapter 2).

The women, on the one hand, lack a coherent aesthetic language to express their pain, but, on the other, they create new forms, such as the lone tree above; and they integrate the cultures by combining both Western and traditional aesthetics within a single drawing or statement, as in the following example (see Figure 3, Image 9):

The woman who drew the calligraphy of the words "Beware of bad people" explained that she is scared of the "bad" youths in her neighborhood and she feels that many dangers exist outside her home.

In this example, the traditional form contains a modern message. Another type of integration is created between traditional form and modern content: This content is written in Hebrew, thus connecting to the Hebrew-Israeli reality of the external culture, but in a traditional calligraphic style.

G. Images as Narrative Triggers

After the women had completed their picture or craft, the finished projects were laid out in a group exhibition at their creators' feet. This method established a direct connection between the individual artwork and the woman who created it (as compared to images in galleries or in the media that are disconnected from their creators). This type of display created an inner circle of images and an outer circle of the women looking at these images. Each woman explained her image, and others could ask questions or comment, while at the same time the circle of images also constituted a group exhibition. The following analyses will focus on the levels of meaning and interpretation of images that this discussion initiated.

H. Gaps between Verbal and Visual Information

The images and their explanations portrayed potentially opposing ideas that together conveyed a complex multifaceted interpretation that was a type of dramatic narrative in which the image and the words were part of the explanation (see Figure 1, Image 6). For example, the image of the traditional tent in Figure 1, Image 4 was in contrast to the modern woman who described it (see Figure 3, Image 10):

The young woman who created this image arrived at the women's center with no traditional head covering, tight fitting clothes, and a large Star of David necklace (a symbol of Jewish culture). Her explanation was that she liked the traditional Bedouin culture best and imagined that it would be nice to have lived in that time, although she personally viewed her own life as very modern. The contrast between the woman's visual message of her clothes and the visual message of her artwork reveals the multiple layers of reality that constitute her life and world. The tent was drawn decoratively, as if to symbolize or evoke a traditional world rather than portraying a real or specific tent.

The young women did not see her own life as only traditional, rejecting modern culture, or only modern, rejecting traditional culture; instead, she was a member of both. Indeed, this woman drew a traditional image of a tent but was dressed in a modern manner; she integrated these two opposing "visuals" through a narrative that describes both sides of the issue. Similarly, the thin blonde woman previously drawn was in extreme contrast to the physical body of the creator, who was a large, traditionally dressed woman (see Figure 2, Images 9 and 10).

44 *Art as a Speech Act from the Margins*

Another example is how the image of the sheikh and wife dolls (Figure 2, Images 9 and 10) were visually innocent, but the creator's explanation was how she ignored her husband by saying "yes" but continuing to do what she wanted to do. Similarly, in the example of the image of the traditional woman holding hands with the "modern" woman (see Figure 2, Image 14), the artist explained that the modern women were pulling the traditional women in their direction—a fact that was left out of the text. It seemed that, while the image was static and thus used to convey cultural values, the discussion around the image in a closed circle of women was allowed to be subversive, adding an additional layer to the understanding of the images.

I. Group Definition of the Content

The group discussing the images can also redefine the creators' meanings, as in the example of the house defined as a black circle (see Figure 3, Image 11).

One woman in the group could not find the words to define what she meant by the black circle she drew. A friend sitting next to her explained that she saw the black circle as representing the sadness of the artist caused by the tight living conditions in her family. The black circle symbolized the constriction she felt living at home. As the friend explained, "I think you are drawing that you feel closed in a circle you can't get out of because there are so many people in your small house." The artist nodded in agreement.

This interaction can also oppose the creators' meanings as a confrontation with the original meaning of the image, as exemplified in the following excerpt of text:

P 4: [Kept starting to make woman figurines out of clay and then ruining them.] "I can't make a woman; I can't find the energy to hold the bits together."

P 2: "We will help you. We are your friends. We know it's hard for you, but it will be okay."

P 4: "No, you don't understand."

P 2: "We do understand; we all feel like that sometimes. You should tell us about your feelings."

P 4: "Thank you; I appreciate your kindness."

After this conversation, Participant 4 began joining her clay bits together, and, while the other women were talking about their images, she started to combine the bits together into a ball.

P 2: "I see it has helped put the bits of clay back together."

Pain and Resilience as Seen in the Compositional Elements 45

The emotional support and the distancing of the image also created a new, more enabling interpretation of reality. This is also apparent in the following discussion of an image previously described:

P 1: "I did a picture of a fish in the sea the fish is alone, because I feel alone."
P 2: "But you are not alone; we are here with you."
P 1: "No, no, I am alone. Also tomorrow I have a driving test and I am very scared to fail. I cannot afford to take it again. I am full of fears today."
P 2: "The fish here is alone, in this picture; but in the sea, there are many fish, like in this group."

The meaning of the image was renegotiated from alone to together.

P 1: "I am like the sea. When there are big winds, I am angry and sad. And when it's calm, I am happy. Today the sea is calm."
P 2: "I don't think that people are like the sea. People can control how they react and how they feel."

This is a way of redefining "what we see" according to a shared cultural context and thus opposing that cultural context, as in the next example that creates a new definition of a woman as strong rather than weak (see Figure 3, Image 12).

P 6: [Making a small cow out of clay]. "A woman is like a cow. If the woman gives milk, it's looked after, but after it doesn't give milk, it's discarded." [She bursts into tears].
P 3: [Quickly making a horse]. "A woman is not like a cow; she is like a horse—strong, and carrying burdens on her back."
P 1: [Making a flower]. "A woman is delicate and pretty like a flower."
P 4: [Making an ashtray]. "The ashtray is like women—a container; An older woman is like an ashtray, like an empty container, when she cannot have children." [She cries].
P 3: "You must fill yourself up, by going to learn, learning to read and write, doing activities, going for a walk with the children in the evening. You must not let yourself despair."

These examples demonstrate that the women do constantly struggle and fight back rather than, as they are often portrayed, passively accepting their hardships. This dynamic of resistance is hidden in the image, composition, or explanation such as climbing up hill to study, struggling to negotiate a driver's license, or learning to manage money.

Women who preferred to create craft objects also explained the process as empowering:

A woman stated that she wanted to take her picture home, that she was proud of it, and wanted to decorate her house, as she could not afford to purchase decorations for her home.

At the end of the session, one woman described the pride she felt in her brooch and how she wanted to wear it to a wedding the following day where she would tell everyone that she made it. She stated that it was not only the cost of the brooch that she was proud of, as it was relatively cheap, but that she made it and that everyone at the wedding would acknowledge her skill.

This example points to the fact that, although the woman is very poor, she also searches for a sense of accomplishment and recognition from peers and her society, which can be achieved by creating things. This group had a sale of their craft objects and managed to make some money. They are also considering setting up a small craft business.

We've seen that impoverished Bedouin women are under the power of different and often opposing groups, including Bedouin men, the Israeli state, Jewish men and women, and middle-class Bedouin women.

This type of indirect resistance toward power holders permeated the process of image making, the images themselves, and the discussion and observation of the images. We saw in the previous section how the women used "wishes" to indirectly ask for physical things such as houses as well as metaphors and symbols to indirectly ask for protection or freedom. Within the process of image making, the women in the group did not show up when the craft materials they asked for were not provided; thus silently and indirectly demanding what they wanted.

Ways that the Bedouin women resist power through images have been shown. However, the ways that power holders—such as myself, the researcher—use images to express our power were also apparent in all stages of the work.

As previously described, on the level of process, at the negotiation stage of the research, one of the art groups did not want to draw but rather, asked for more crafts materials; however, the social worker who worked with the group claimed that because the Bedouin women only do crafts they are "not creative" and thus needed to learn expressive art, although they requested a crafts orientation. While I disagreed with her verbally, I also "forgot" to use the crafts material we brought to make fabric dolls at the women's request, instead staying with expressive art, which is more familiar to me. However, the women did not all turn up to the next meeting, so I, the researcher, had to shift to what they wanted in order to continue the research.

Thus, the organization of image-based workshops and the use of images, as a non power-infused area (as compared to welfare aid, for example), was more flexible to enable negotiation but also showed power struggles. At the same time, we see that the use of images did not disseminate power struggles, but rather emulated them, as well as creating a flexible and indirect space within which to negotiate them. For example, the social worker wanted the women to learn "real expressive art"; she labeled them as uncreative because they "only" embroidered.

This was apparent with the Bedouin social worker of the group, who was present in the drawing sessions and who stated that the women's art flooded her with their pain and created disorientation about how to lead the group. This was a new perspective she had not encountered in her previous work with the women, whom she often experienced as manipulatively helpless. On the other hand, the images were described by the social worker as creating enough distance from the women's stress to be able to understand what they wanted, or to "get the whole picture" of what they needed. She realized that they were lonely and needed a space of their own: Usually she could not react effectively, as the flooding of words and tears made her feel overwhelmed or caused her to disengage. The symbols contain both the creator and the observers' emotions.

As shown in the above description, the images were also effective in influencing power holders, such as the group social worker, who understood their wishes through these images and helped them organize a clubhouse where they could have activities for their children. The clubhouse offers them a space to be together that counteracts the isolation of being alone in a house and the difficulty they have with their children returning to collective female spaces. Thus, the group explanation of images became an effective speech act which enabled the women to influence power holders, to communicate their needs to their social worker, and to change their environment. It assisted in building a concrete and symbolic space for them within the community.

Section 2
Using Images from a Socially Contextualized Perspective within Social Research and Practice

The images created by the Bedouin women were analyzed on the level of content and form. The content analysis conveyed the experience of the cultural transition from a nomadic lifestyle to an urban sedentary lifestyle in townships, living in poverty, and multiple levels of marginalization (Al-Ataana, 1993, 2002; Cwikel, 2002; Lewando-Hundt, 1976, 1978; Meir, 2005; Perez, 2001). Understanding the experience of this transition enables researchers to capture the history of the rapid transition to modernity that the Bedouin culture, as a whole, is undergoing, from the standpoint of marginalized women (Lazreg, 1994; Lawler, 2002).

The aesthetic analysis, specifically, and the aesthetic tactics of mapping, wishing, symbolizing, and integrating personal experience through the use of both new and traditional forms embody the ways that the women respond to the social context of their lives. This experience includes representing pain with symbols, which is a way that the women use indirectly to try to enter the Westernization process, as well as attempting to take back their spaces and resources. They use ways that enable them to integrate rather than split the two cultures and a way that enables them to redefine their identity within this shifting context.

The two analyses of form and content acknowledge the Bedouin women's experience as objective or socially constructed, and simultaneously as subjective; that is, emanating from the inside and the outside. The innovation of using images as data is that they can portray these two levels, the content and the experience of that content; in other words, simultaneously how it "is," but also how it "feels" and how it could be made better, creating a complex and multifaceted vision as a database and as an intervention.

The claim of this book is that both levels, form and content, are relevant to all of the fields in the social sciences that utilize images. This relevance will be demonstrated in the following section of the book, and its implications for arts-based research, art therapy, group empowerment, social change, and conflict negotiation will be outlined in later chapters.

These concepts will now be applied as a theoretical model to different fields in the social sciences that use images: to therapy and art empowerment, which tend to focus on compositional type of analyses, and to arts-based research and art as social action, which tend to focus on content-based analyses.

This section of the book will outline an overall theoretical and methodological model for using images from a social perspective, showing how the same images can be utilized for research, therapy, empowerment, and social action. In each of these areas, case studies will be presented to help generalize and illustrate these directions.

5 Using Images in Research from a Social Perspective

A. Background on Images within Research

There is an explosion of image-based research and practice methodology in the social sciences. Researchers in education, psychology, geography, political science, art therapy, and other areas all include images in their studies. In all of these areas, however, images are often illustrative of and less dominant than words: Each area stays within the boundaries of its specific field and subserves images to them, rather than looking laterally at how other disciplines are using images and taking their inherent characteristics into account. Within art therapy, for example, the wish to become a psychologically accepted field focuses on proving the effectiveness of using images from a psychological perspective, rather than on gaining a social understanding of what the images convey (Johnson, 1999). This includes a neurological perspective and universal projective tests. Similarly, arts-based research, often rather romantically, assumes that images are a "deep" or inherent personal statement rather than a construction in the context of a reaction to a specific social reality. From this perspective, images are assumed to be therapeutic also in research contexts (Knowles & Cole, 2008; Levy, 1997; Sclater, 2003). Both of these directions, arts-based research and art therapy research, tend to remove images from social reality and limit the understanding of images as renderings of universal neurological and unconscious or, alternatively, subjective phenomenological levels of experience (Burns, 1987; O'Callaghan, 2008; Silver, 2001, 2005).

Conversely, within visual anthropology and visual culture, images are often understood as blueprints or illustrations of social processes, disregarding the ability of images to transform self and culture (Emerson & Smith, 2000; Huss, 2009a,b; Mason, 2002).

Within the case study of Bedouin women in Section 1, the aim of the research was to introduce a social analytical prism that included both the anthropological and the phenomenological perspectives described above. Images are defined as constructed by, but also as reacting to, a specific social reality and its power structures. The social reality was expressed in the content level, while the reactions to oppression, marginalization, trauma, and cultural transition were captured in the aesthetic structure of images. This analysis combines humanistic or subjective as well as social or contextualized prisms of understanding. This is similar to Mahon's (2000) concept of "embedded aesthetics," which argues that the aesthetic product is not "inherent from within" but always part of broader social contexts, which both transform and are transformed by the art product, and around which there is always a power struggle over different cultural meanings. The question is what mechanisms of representation and explanation enable this? As compared to Rose's (1988) concept of a single theoretical glasses through which we understand an image, this book claims that we must learn to wear multiple glasses, or to shift perspectives, so as to create a rounded but tentative analysis that captures complex multifaceted experience.

B. Mapping Experience into Space: Challenging Verbal Narratives

First, we've seen how creating an image of an experience converts that experience from an abstract verbal concept into a concrete spatial object. We've seen how this translation defines the relative size and physical distance between objects, in terms of subject, background, and interaction between the elements that create the narrative or content of the image (Huss & Cwikel, 2005). However, because the empty page is a symbolic as well as a concrete space, the space between objects—in terms of the overall composition and relationship between elements such as line, color, contour, and size—becomes a symbolic depiction of the conceptual and emotional distance between people in relation to each other and in relation to the abstract things that they want. This was shown in the present case study in terms of the distances between men, women, and children and of the difficulty of obtaining access to inside and outside spaces and mobility to move within and between them. This definition of identity and social marginalization through spatial concepts is also exemplified in the following research: Alush (2012), in her research on how impoverished at-risk teenage girls living in a well-known city slum experience their neighborhood, asked them to create photographs of the spaces that they live in and that they are connected to. The young girls photographed the areas that they defined as scary and "trashed," as well as the areas that conveyed a sense of community and positive childhood memories. The girls claimed that while the trash of the area was disturbing for them, they, themselves, had also "trashed" the neighborhood, as described in the following (see Figure 4):

> Look at all the trash! It's disgusting, but our house is very clean. I have to clean it—don't get me wrong, at home I help to clean all the

time. I wash the floor every day but, outside, I throw stuff on the floor as well.

The "trashed" surroundings that the girls live in when revealed to them in images, enables reflection and dialogue with the duality that has internalized the trash and the trashing, as part of the young girls' identity that both cleans and trashes at the same time. This representation enables a spatial depiction of the marginalization experience that is not locked into verbal abstractions. The spatial organization of the images shows the context of the girls' lives through symbols, composition, shape, size, and overall organization, rather than through verbal abstractions such as "low self-esteem." This approach destabilizes existing psychological narratives that often hide cultural and social marginalization.

For example, rather than being labeled in psychological terms such as *displaying delinquent behavior, lacking impulse control*, or *acting out*, the girls are shown to be reacting to the complex limitations of the spaces in which they live that they both clean and trash. In other words, the use of spatial concepts challenges existing knowledge structures, such as identity, in terms of spatial relations rather than in terms of abstractions, pointing to the use of art as an indigenous and in this case feminist research method that "decolonizes" academic-psychological universalist concepts (Tuhiwai-Smith, 1999). On this level, research that relates to concrete space becomes a type of indigenous and feminist research method that destabilizes patriarchal and hegemonic power discourses. The types of spaces that bodies move within are shown in all of the images of the Bedouin women shown previously and in the relationship between character and background as a fresh way to explore identity (Abu-Said & Champagne, 2005; Brington & Likes, 1999; Dallow, 2007; Dwairy, 2004; Eisner, 1997; Emmerson & Smith, 2000; Foster, 2007; Harrington, 2004; Huss, Alhozeyel, & Marcus, 2012; Mohanty, 2003; Moor, 1997; Piquemal, 2005; Reid, 1993; Soja, 1989; Tuhiwai-Smith, 1999).

In his book on political geography, Soja (1989) writes, "Class struggle must encompass and focus upon the vulnerable point of the production of space, the reassertion of space in critical social theory" (p. 92).

In all countries, but maybe especially in conflicted countries, such as Israel, where this research took place, space is always a political issue. Thus, when women spatially depict their private experiences of relationships, these depictions become politicized. On this level, images are shown to destabilize the parameters of verbal research itself and to point directly to the lack of spaces and to the impact of "trashed" spaces and of lack of spaces on identity (Huss, 2007, 2008, 2012).

C. Images as Symbols to Express Pain

Campbell (1999) describes how lived experiences become meaningful through coherent narratives that use symbolic productions. Wolfgang (2006) describes symbols as addressing the specific needs of people in specific times and then being exchanged for new symbols as times change (Huss, 2008).

How do images of symbols capture these belief systems? In the Bedouin women's images described previously, the symbols that were drawn, such as the birds, ants, or tree, all represented a complex situation beyond a single metonymic definition. The symbols contain both cognition and emotion and allow for a complex understanding of the women's experience in the context of a specific social reality, including how they feel, how they understand it, how the social context creates and reacts to the problem, and also how they cope. Multiple types of information are transmitted through a symbol.

Another contribution of symbols to research is that intense emotions, such as pain, are hard to capture within research because they are too painful to be verbalized and addressed directly in a research context. Images help distance these emotions by projecting them onto the page. The emotion is also contained within a symbol, which is another way to distance the pain. Images of symbols use metaphors of painful emotions that also create distance. For example, in the Bedouin women's images, birds seeking food, an isolated ant, a tree swaying in the wind, images of nature, are used to distance human emotions, and to help to access experiences in research that are often too painful to verbalize directly. The literature on trauma reactions shows how intensely painful experiences are often caught in images rather than in words, because the pain and magnitude of trauma break down former meaning based on a stable sense of reality, which has been shattered. This level of pain cannot be cognitively processed and verbalized (Sarid & Huss, 2010; van Der Kolk, Hopper, & Osterman, 2001). By starting with an image, the pain is given a primary form that is also controlled and distanced. This process can become a starting point for exploring emotional as well as cognitive understandings of this pain within a research context (Huss & Cwikel, 2008a).

In the following example, a group of Israeli Jewish research participants explored the meaning of death of a loved one, an intensely painful situation (Schechter, 2012). One woman described her husband's sudden death as "blue."

> I drew death as blue. I searched for the right blue rays; death for me is blue, a bright color. When Yossi died, a blue light emanated from him; I can't explain it, from his eyes, it covered him. So I said, "Ok, he's dead, he's surrounded in blue ... a blue light, that's how I remember it."

In this example, the color blue becomes a metaphor for death which is not fully explained, but verbalizing "blue" rather than "death" enables the woman to talk about death, which is an experience that is difficult to express due to her pain and loss and also due to the social taboo of discussing death in Western culture. Thus, using images becomes a way to discuss pain that is both internally painful and also a social taboo within a given culture. In other words, images help to access an experience for which there may not be words within a specific culture, to focus on the relationship between personal pain and social construction or treatment of pain, which can decontextualize intense emotions into a specific social reality or background (Willmott, 2000).

Once the symbol is drawn, then words can be found to explain the image, for the painful experiences that are described in the symbol and distanced from the socially unacceptable or meaning-shattering experience—words that are based on the characteristics of the symbol rather than on the direct emotion. This process helps the participant to verbalize and define the experience for herself and for others from a safe distance. The cognitive process of defining or explaining a symbol or image that is a broad type of information helps to define gaps between emotional and cognitive understandings (Furth, 1998; Jung, 1974; Riley, 1997; Save & Nuutinen, 2003). In other words, drawing or capturing visual symbols enables a new perspective of the emotion to be reached and becomes a meeting place between cognitive versus emotional reality. This enables the participant to locate the pain within a socially constructed reality, rather than as an inherent part of the participant. For example, the Bedouin woman who portrayed herself as a tree struggling in the wind but trying to stay strong, defined the wind as her poverty, and herself as strong, rather than the opposite. The overall presentation of a woman shifted from that of weakness as exemplified in the image of a discarded ashtray to that of strength as exemplified in an image of a weak cow turning into a strong horse: The discussion was grounded in these images rather than in abstract psychological or social concepts (see chapters 3 and 4).

In the following research example, a social worker draws an image of her fear in a war situation. The social worker described how some social workers were sent with ambulance crews to places where rockets were actively falling to help people suffering from shock and other stress reactions (Huss et al., 2011; see Figure 10).

> I symbolized my experience as a person torn apart in the middle with endless demands made on her—fragmenting her thin empty body—she has nothing to give anyone ... she is so scared.... We were mostly needed to help put wounded people and people suffering from anxiety attacks into the ambulances. We were expected to talk to them and to calm them down. But it was terrifying for me to

56 *Using Images from a Socially Contextualized Perspective*

be there, to endanger my life. Also, my mother criticized me for leaving my kids and risking my life in the middle of the war, all for my job. I drew how fragmented and flooded by different demands I feel.

The explanation of the symbols thus reveals the fragmented experience and connects it to a specific social reality rather than defining her as an anxious or fragmented person. This process provides a social, rather than a pathological context for understanding pain. Rather than defining her as "traumatized," it shows the price of a social phenomenon such as war on the individual and the difficulty of her situation as a woman and social worker.

D. Images as Indirectly Expressing Social Taboos

The above types of traumatic and painful experiences are part of the reality of marginalized groups that have often undergone different forms of loss, including immigration, war, violence, sexual abuse, intense poverty, and natural and manmade disasters, on top of the pervasive stress of ongoing poverty that initiates some of the above (Huss, Sarid, & Cwikel, 2010; see Figure 8).

In the following example, a group of survivors of sexual abuse drew images of their experience of incest, which is both an inner trauma but also a socially taboo subject. The victim is often blamed as somehow responsible, while the perpetrator is not severely punished (Huss, Kacen, & Hirschen, 2012; Zeligman & Solomon, 2004). The color black was used in their images, and the word *black* was used by all of the participants instead of directly naming the sexual abuse that they had all experienced: In Figure 8, Image 4, a woman described her experience of sexual abuse as a "blackness" that is constantly there, even in good times (Huss et al., 2012).

The color black became a group symbol that enabled the women to explore facets of their experience (see Figure 8, Image 1). Interestingly, in Figure 8.1 we see how the black sits at the center of the image, as internalized by the woman while the world is drawn as colorful. However, black words cover the surroundings, stating that this is a bad world. The experience is internalized but through the image, also reconstructed socially. Discussing the experience in terms of images, without naming the sexual abuse, which is a socially stigmatized concept, allows these different facets of the experience to be verbalized and explored, which produces a dialogue with the experience that has been researched. Interestingly, we see that both death and sexual abuse are described through colors alone, as if these experiences cannot yet be more clearly defined into a shape with specific contours because they are so painful.

Images, as dialogues with the pain, capture the reactions to the experience as well as the experience itself, in other words, the defenses and coping methods as shown in the following example.

In Figure 8, Image 2 the woman drew boxes over the page, and explained her experience of incest as inaccessible to her: "these boxes are like those cardboard boxes in the supermarket that fall open if you put too much into them."

However, in her next image (Figure 8, Image 3) she described a metonym of the "not helping" that related more directly to her experience of sexual abuse. She explained that the hands were "helping"; however, another participant confronted her statement, pointing to her deference as captured in the image: "The hands are not helping, they could also be understood as attacking ... the hands are attacking and no one is helping" (see also analyses, Chapter 9).

Through the images and symbols, such as the box, the color black, and the hands, the painful experience was made accessible, but it was also socially contextualized into a reality that enabled it to be defined as research, rather than being defined as an illness, such as PTSD or dissociation; and this enables us to understand an experience within its social reality that also constructed it.

However, images can also show gaps between cognition and emotion. In the following research example, the gap between the socially constructed theories and the difficult emotional experience of social work students meeting people suffering from extreme poverty and hunger was shown through the students' images of poverty (Kaufman, Huss, & Segal-Engelchin, 2011). Although the students intellectually understood poverty and food insecurity as a systemic and socially constructed problem, due to neocapitalism and the fall of the welfare state (Alcock, 1997), the images they drew of the people they met showed that they emotionally experienced extremely poor and hungry people as arousing anger and pity. They defined them as helpless, ineffective, and in some way blamed them for their extreme poverty. This was described in the following example as a "hole" that pulls people in (see Figure 5):

> I drew food insecurity as a type of hole that pulls everything—physical, emotional, spiritual and personal contents—into it; a hole that is hard to climb out of if you fall into it. When I reach homes that are socio-economically poor, I am always offered cola and sweets, and the children say they didn't know they had that at home; why aren't they allowed to drink it? And the kids, when you meet them at school, they all the time talk about food.

The image enables the researcher to understand what the students feel, rather than what they think. Discussing symbols enables researchers to explore the gap between individual and social constructs of reality in processed groups, such as students, a gap that words often hide.

Interestingly, in contrast to this example, the Bedouin women expressed the socially accepted narrative in images, while their explanations held the culturally unacceptable explanations: This contradiction may be because the image is perceived as a more concrete document, whereas the discussion in the group is only between women; in other words, the image, or its explanation, can hold personal emotional or cognitive social explanations.

E. Images as Capturing Hybrid Cultural Realities

As stated throughout the book, images and symbols are not only personal symbols but are also created in the context of a specific society and in dialogue with that society. For example, the color blue was used by the woman to describe her husband's death; in Israel, the blue is connected to spiritual and Zionist elements, a color on the Israeli flag, and the concept that one has to die for one's country embedded within Zionist ideology. Similarly, her use of an undefined shape of blue can be understood as part of the aesthetics of drawing an abstract shape or color within Western art (Hills, 2001). Similarly, the Bedouin women used symbols of trees and nature, which are accepted forms for conveying emotion within Islamic aesthetics (Irving, 1997). These cultural understandings would be lost if the symbol were only understood in the frame of a personal or universal explanation (2008).

At the same time, culturally embedded meanings are dynamic, shifting, and multifaceted. If we assume that people constantly reinterpret culture and use cultural symbols to reinterpret experience, then understanding the social context of the aesthetic and symbolic elements in an image becomes a way to understand how the participant shifts, integrates, or splits different cultural realities. For example, the above-described Bedouin women utilized traditional symbolic contents in new compositional forms, such as a single tree alone, or a crying tree, or modern rather than symbolic depictions of nature (see Chapters 3 and 4).

The multiple levels of image making and explaining enable researchers to see how people integrate or map out their different cultural realities. Images are an effective medium by which to understand different cultural realities; for example, researching populations that are transitioning from a collective to an individualistic society, from rural to urban living, or from a position of poverty; that is, populations that cannot "afford" a coherent and single cultural form. Thus, images are a useful research tool for global and postmodern society, where identity is split and integrated in different ways. As Lippard (1990) states:

Hybrid and emotionally complex stories derived from both tradition and experience, old-new stories, challenge the pervasive 'master narratives' that would contain them. (p. 57)

One of a group of Bedouin children living in a township drew a billboard with a woman wearing a Western wedding dress (image not shown) with exposed hair, which is culturally sanctioned because it's wedding attire. Next to this image was the mosque, which represents the Islamic doctrine that requires women to cover their hair and body in public. The child showed how, within his understanding, seemingly opposing traditional and Western conceptions live side by side within the same picture. This creates a new and hybrid cultural statement; the image is a good place to show not only that people do integrate different cultures, but also how people integrate different cultural realities.

F. Using Images as a Trigger for Different Narratives

Image making and then explanation by the image maker or with peers were shown, in the above-described Bedouin case study, to create multiple levels of interpretation by the research participants. First, the image itself is an interpretation of reality. Second, the explanation of the image becomes another interpretive level; and finally, the dialogue with others around the image becomes the third level of interpretation (Huss, 2007).

The analysis becomes a type of action research process in that the different levels of interpretation intensify the research participants' voices but also create a transformation in meanings. In other words, visual depiction helps not only to define experience, but also to redefine experience as meanings are gradually transformed. We saw this in relation to the case study of the Bedouin woman who redefined another woman from weak to strong through her explanations of images. Similarly, the social work students described above revealed that the culture of social work education did not take into account the emotional impact of poverty on social workers who relate directly to these people. Similarly, the women who had experienced death and incest started to define and verbalize an experience that is both deeply painful and culturally taboo through the use of images in a more enabling and socially connected form.

The group context for understanding images can further intensify this shift in meanings within a group of participants that share the same reality. This can be a way to create a type of focus group that self-defines a group's understanding of a specific social reality and expands their understanding of shared experiences.

In the following example, a group of social workers was asked to creatively render genograms of their families by adding images and symbols to the gender map (Huss & Cwikel, 2008c). One woman noticed that all the women in her family worked in the helping professions (Figure 8, Image 1) whereas all the men worked in scientific and engineering-related professions. This pattern included herself and her new husband. She had majored in science but, in compliance with the described pattern, later chose to retrain as a social worker. The participant pointed out that the two divorced women in her family had careers in science; and, therefore, she thought that perhaps "it really was a mistake for women to try to enter a 'man's' profession.'" While this explanation accepts the familial and gendered message, the participant had covered her genogram with a "prison" grid, creating a visual rendering that expressed her anger toward the gendered roles that she had apparently accepted.

In another example of an image-based genogram (Figure 8, Image 2), a woman described how all the men in her family were quiet like fish and all the women were verbal like butterflies. However, she was like a fish in her temperament and very quiet. This complicated her gendered role and was her explanation for her difficulty in finding a husband. Other group members, however, described different animals, such as a cat, that is quiet but very expressive and feminine, challenging her social understanding.

This image illustrates the use of symbols to resist and to transform social meanings (women as butterflies and men as fish, or women in social work and men in science). This illustrates the next point, that images also enable human beings to imagine and to concretize solutions, which is an area that is elusive to capture in research about reality rather than imagination.

G. Images as Envisaging Solutions

As stated above, once the issue has been defined, then images can also envisage solutions because they do not have to represent reality. This use of images has the potential to be a method for strength-based understandings of how people, rather than experts, conceptualize, cope with and solve painful social realities (Kisthardt, 1997; Lazarus, 1994; Masten, 2001). For example, we saw how the Bedouin women suggested many solutions to their self-defined problems, including being outside together, ignoring but placating husbands, "filling oneself up" instead of being a discarded ashtray, imagining planting one's own garden, and having one's own house. The wishes that they expressed were solutions to the deprivation that they experienced.

In the following research example, images were used to access visions of self-fulfillment of a group of unemployed at-risk women (Magos, 2012). This image (Figure 7) is explained by the artist this way:

> I made the tree large; it symbolizes me, so I remember to put myself in the middle of my life. That's what holding down a job means to

me, putting myself in the middle ... and looking after that tree—giving it water and—it's my responsibility to look after my own tree.

The woman's image challenged stereotypes of poor women as being concerned only with the basic levels of survival or self-actualization, and it showed a complex and rich spectrum of definitions of self-fulfillment as defined by Maslow (1970). The image is concerned with self-respect (Brington & Lykes, 1996; Miller, 1996).

Figure 7, Image 2 shows a woman standing and talking at her desk at work and also points to the importance of having a voice as being above the money earned in a job; in other words, self-expression is a more important value for this woman then having a job:

> I want to say what I really want to say ... I drew me standing, talking behind a desk at work; to talk, to say what I want, to reach out to others; you know, I don't want to be someone who never talks, because then I can't find people to help me or who could love me.

These types of images enable researchers to learn how people conceptualize and solve problems, to see what their visions and dreams are, and to gain an insight into the problems. Mullen describes this as "us[ing] the imagination not only to examine how things are, but also how they could be" (Mullen, 2003, p. 117). This analysis creates a strength-based methodology for viewing how people cope and solve problems, which is participatory and action-based in nature.

H. Images as Indirect Negotiation with Power-Holders

Another way of understanding images in research, as in transactional analysis, is as transactions with different observers and as constructed as methods to negotiate power with these observers. This understanding creates another analytical prism. The researcher or imagined or real observer of the image is always a representative of a power structure, and so images in research are constructed in relation to these different levels of power (Mahon, 2000).

We have seen, in the case study of the Bedouin women, that indirect resistance toward power holders permeated the process of the Bedouin women's image making and discussion. Images of metaphors and symbols were used to indirectly ask for protection, freedom, space, and mobility; images were also used to compete with and resist the power of Bedouin men and the Jewish state. The women mimicked and emulated the dominant culture, represented by the group leader. Likewise, the above images that the impoverished, unemployed women drew could be seen as a guide to satisfy the social workers in whose groups they met and on whom they were dependent for various funds. Similarly, the young girls who notified the researcher that they trashed their neighborhood, may also be expressing their rebellion against their cultural and social differences to an outsider.

In this chapter, the methodological advantage of using images in research in the social sciences was defined as their ability to concretize context through a spatial medium, as well as their ability to distance painful emotional experiences through symbolizing content. This enables access to intense and painful emotional experiences, which are difficult to discuss directly due to inner defenses or cultural taboos regarding the source of the pain. Additionally, the use of images as a way to access a participant's interpretations and solutions of the events researched was examined. Another direction that was introduced was the use of images to reveal a hybrid cultural experience through the interplay of socially contextualized compositional mechanisms. Finally, the use of images to envisage coping and solutions and to concretize them was discussed (Huss & Cwikel, 2005; Huss, 2010d).

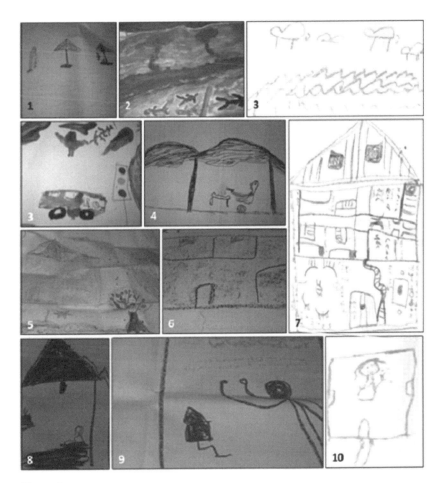

Figure 1

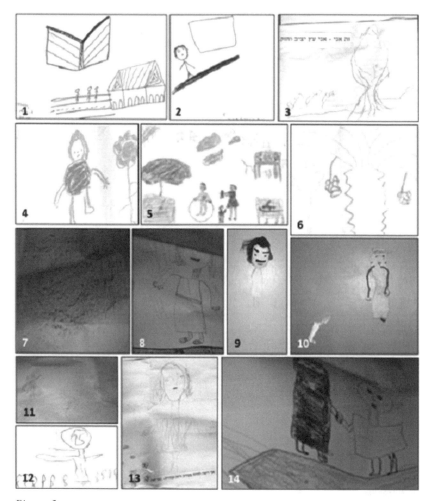

Figure 2

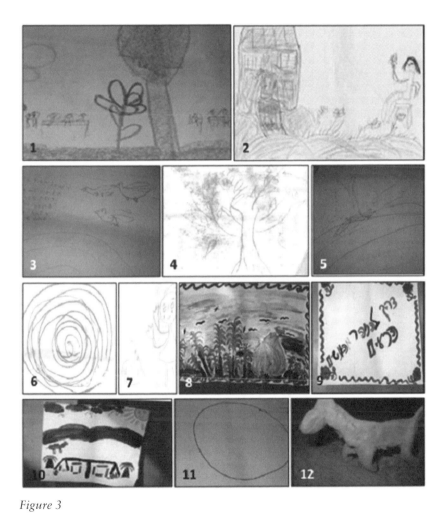

Figure 3

Trashed neighborhood

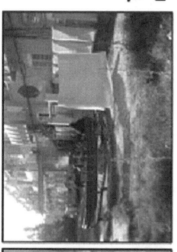 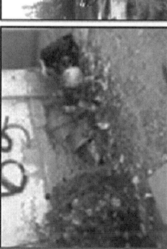

People come and sit and dirt the area, not the mothers of the small children who come to the park of course- but us, we trash it-f we walk to our park now you will smell the trash, and see it, we look after our own houses but we trash the public areas.

Figure 4

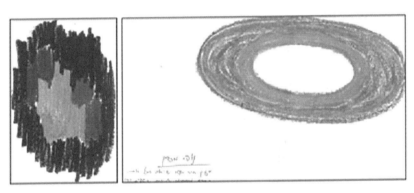

"I drew food insecurity as a type of hole that pulls everything, physical, emotional, spiritual and personal, into it—a hole that is hard to climb out of if you fall into it. When I reach homes that are socio-economically poor, I am always offered cola and sweets, and the children said, they didn't know they had that at home, why aren't they allowed to drink it? And the kids, when you meet them at school, they all the time talk about food."

Figure 5

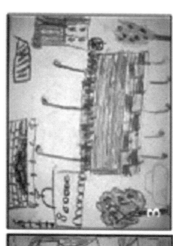
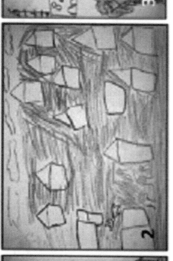
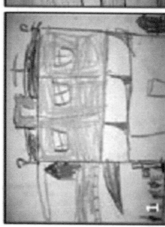

1. Township Here is my big house, with a fence around i.t
2. Village - This is my home, my village.
3. This is our carpet that my mother made and that we eat on every day.

Figure 6

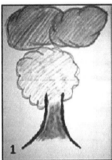 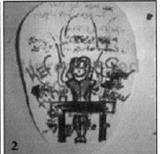 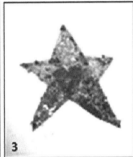

1. "I made the tree large, it symbolizes me, so I remember to put myself in the middle of my life- that's what holding down a job means to me, putting myself in the middle..- and looking after that tree- giving it water and air- it's my responsibility, to look after my own tree".

2. "I want to say what I really want to say... I drew me standing, talking- behind a desk at work- to talk, to say what I want, to reach out to others; you know,. I don't want to be someone who never talks, because then I can't find people to help me or who could love me.. ."

3. "At the beginning I wanted to paint the whole star bright pink, which is happiness, because I finally got a job, and I am so happy, and then I thought, just a minute, it will take time- it's hard work, so I painted it half purple and half pink- to remind myself that it's not going to be easy so I won't be disappointed".

Figure 7

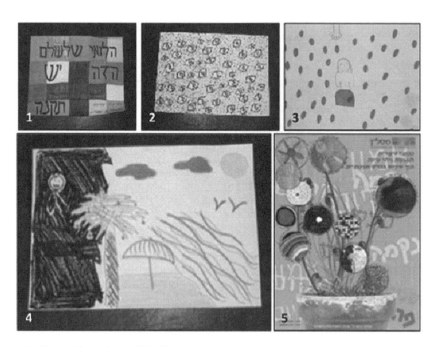

1. If only this world could be fixed.
2. "These boxes are an illusion, they are not helping, they are open, like those cardboard boxes in the supermarket that fall open if you put too much into them".
3. "The hands are not helping, they could also be understood as attacking... the hands are attacking and no one is helping...".
4. "Even when things are good, the black is always there...".
5. We created a poster together - to raise awareness of sexual abuse - it's made up of our personal pictures, but each person is a flower.

Figure 8

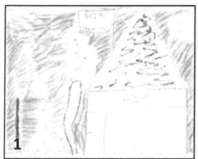 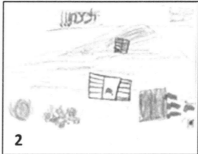

1. "Once there was a boy called Yair and he lived with his family in the Gush, he had a strange feeling, one day, where he heard they would be sent from their homes, he tried to imagine how it would feel, – he asked if only their family would be sent away, and his mother explained that no, they would all go to a big demonstration soon so we demonstrated together, all the families".

2. "My mother is sad, she sits at home, she misses our former home which was by the sea. I drew her wearing an orange kerchief, to give her strength.."

Figure 9

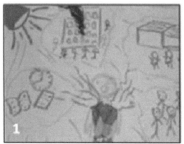 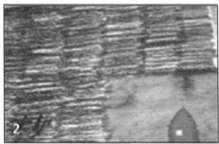

1. "We were mostly needed to help put wounded people and people suffering from anxiety attacks into the ambulances. We were expected to talk to them and to calm them down. But it was terrifying for me to be there, to endanger my life. My mother criticized me for leaving my kids and risking my life in the middle of the war, all for a job. All in all, I feel so fragmented and stressed from these constant and opposing demands".

2. "The fear of being bombed: Loss of a basic sense of safety in one's environment I turned my whole world into a black surround except for my house- as if it's pressing into it. – as if there is nothing except the bombs. This is apparent in the thick, black shaded border".

Figure 10

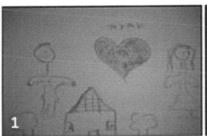 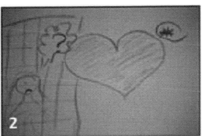

1. "I drew me and my husband to be, and the baby that will be born to us, and this heart is our love. at the end, I added the house we will have".
2. "I drew a young girl with a covered face who is being killed, I think marriage at a young age is like killing your daughter. I will not allow my daughters to get married at a young age. You think marriage is a white dress and a party attention, but it's a relationship, house, children, getting used to a whole new family. I was a young child, I didn't know how to make decisions, and I was irresponsible. I thought marriage would bring freedom, and joy, but I ended up being strangled each time".

Figure 11

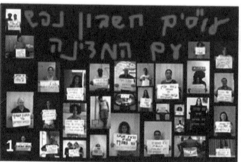 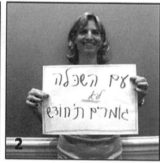

1. Social workers demanding higher pay Social workers demanding pay from the state.
2. A degree does not help finish the month.

Figure 12

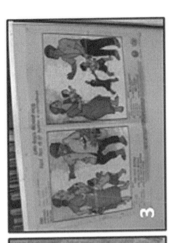
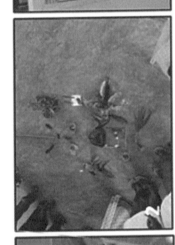
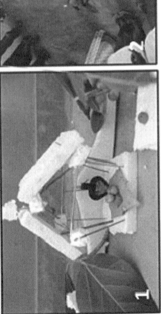

1-2. "Images of Gods that can protect us from a further tsunami.
3. A didactic wall picture for husbands against drinking alcohol.

Figure 13

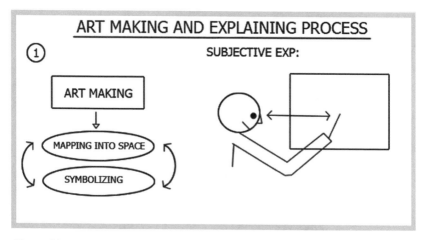

Figure 14

6 Methodological Implications of Using Images within Research

Sullivan (2001) uses the "rope" metaphor to describe the complex, multilayered interaction of art form, with each element of the art process, product, and context all being part of an intertwined rope that forms the art speech act described in the former chapter. Thus, when used as a research method, images include the broad definition of the process of their production and interpretation in addition to the product itself. How does this social rather than fine art perspective translate into the nuts and bolts of using images within research? How are images defined and chosen, how are they created, and how are they explained by their creator and by the researcher? These methodological considerations will together define and guide the role or position that the images will take within the research, as method, subject, data, or end product. Each of these issues and positions will now be delineated so as to provide a methodological map for using images within research contexts from a social context but also phenomenological perspective.

First, the question arises as to whether a population or research issue is suitable for using an image-based method: The methodological advantage of using images to access emotional content, cultural context, and the process of dealing with an issue has been outlined in the previous chapter. From a social perspective, the research concept of verbalizing experience in general, and to strangers such as researchers specifically, is also not always culturally compatible. Symbolic and metaphoric forms of expression, rather than confessional or abstract narrative styles, are cited as more common among poor and rural communities than verbal abstractions (Ben-Ezer, 2002; Bowler, 1997; Reid, 1993; Saulnier, 1996; Spivack, 1993). Similarly, preconceived categories such as questionnaires may be unclear or irrelevant for participants. The use of images can help to convey those forms of expression that are nonverbal and nonexplicit, enabling control of the level of disclosure and direct confrontation with power holders. This is a methodological advantage for research.

A. Definition of Images within Research

Types of images used within research include found artifacts, crafts, contemporary media images, fine art, and self-made images in different forms, such as photography, video, art, diagrams, and imagined images. Consideration of the meaning of these different images for the research participant as well as the relation of the image to the subject of the research should influence the choice of image. This can include the spectrum between ready-made images, such as projective pictures or photographs, or self-defined images, such as photographs, drawings. or diagrams. Alternatively, imagined images can be used, such as those used in guided imagery or images transposed within verbal discussion (O'Callaghan, 2008).

The cultural connotations of images can be learned from the research participant prior to the research: For example, we saw in the Bedouin case study that the use of traditional art forms alone would have been a way of stereotyping a group into using traditional aesthetics that are not fully relevant to them. Conversely, enforcing only Western images was not a solution. The women themselves defined a wish to integrate both types, learning Western-type crafts as well as using traditional crafts. This demanded the combination of two types of information: anthropological understanding but also phenomenological understanding of the meanings of a specific type of image for research participants. For example, is it permitted to draw human figures or the figure of God? Which images are sacred, and which are shameful? This can include both the end product and the process of their creation. Rose's (1988) definitions of the visualizations or cultural lenses through which we observe images needs to be taken into account when choosing a ready-made image as a trigger for projection and discussion. From a cultural perspective, projective cards and images, such as those used in psychology (Silver, 2005), usually contain Western fairytale images such as fairies, goblins, princesses, and so forth. These images and concepts may be unfamiliar to people from non-Western cultures. Issues of "high" versus "low" images (e.g., the Mona Lisa as "high art") have different cultural connotations for different people. For example, in Lalush's research (Lallush, 2012), described in an earlier chapter, which involved young girls photographing the slum areas where they live, the medium of photography was chosen as a "grown-up" medium that would not cause frustration for the young girls as might have been the case if they had used drawing. It would not make them feel childish. It also suited the research question of how the surroundings are experienced.

Another type of use of images to elicit information is undertaken automatically by many social practitioners. The use of visual cues to enhance meaning for social practitioners when researching a client is an inherent part of their work, as described by a social worker:

I remember going for a home visit to an old man who refused to talk. I saw a huge picture of his deceased wife of five years on the wall—that was all there was on the wall—and I started talking about that, as it explained everything. (Huss, 2012, p. 6)

In other words, the limits of the image are also a consideration. In Ben-Israel's study (2012) of an extremist religious area in Israel, he became aware of many murals in the settlement as he went to interview people and decided to focus on them as an additional data level.

Another type of image can be one that is not seen but talked about—as a metaphor in an interview for example—or in visualizations. Imagined images are considered identical in neurological terms to created images. In other words, an imagined image, as compared to an image that is physically seen, arouses the same emotions and reactions (O'Callaghan, 2008; Sarid & Huss, 2010).

Self-made images have the advantage of allowing observation of the process of creating the image. However, the different methods and materials also have social connotations, such as the quality of art materials or the social understanding of the process of creating an image. For example, use of art materials or images with adults that are commonly used by children can be interpreted as lack of respect for an adult, and this perceived insult can impact the image-making process. Conversely, sophisticated techniques or materials can be intimidating for nonartists, and experiencing image making as something one is not good at can make the process uncomfortable and thus also influence the type of image created.

To exemplify the different role of image making within different cultures, an art teacher working with Bedouin children told me how he had asked children to draw a picture of a tree that they see in their village; the children had gone directly to the person who is considered to be the best artist in the village and asked him to draw the tree.

This collective versus individualistic understanding of images, which is based on product rather than process, means that art as self-expression is not culturally familiar to many people. Marginalized groups who are used to being diagnosed and defined by others will often rightly assume that any art they create will be used to diagnose them. In the past, this type of diagnosis has resulted in intense outcomes such as psychiatric labels or removal of children from their homes. Indeed, images can have legal reverberations (Rubins, 2001; Silver, 2001, 2005). Further, different art materials have specific characteristics that influence the type of image created. This influence can depend on whether the material is familiar to the creator, if it has cultural connotations, and also on the inherent characteristics of the material. For example, pencils can create diagrams better than paint, which can create looser types of images with a focus on color; collage overcomes the problem of drawing, but the

66 *Using Images from a Socially Contextualized Perspective*

types of materials used in the collage will also define the types of images created. In Schechter's (2012) research on images of death described in an earlier chapter, and in the group of sexual abuse survivors, different materials were offered so that each participant could choose the level of control or degree of color (Rubin, 2001).

Overall, an understanding of the art process and materials as impacting the content points to the need to understand the meanings of different materials and types of images in the context of a specific group of research participants. Images are always part of a cultural construct and thus are not neutral, and their social implications must be taken into account in the structuring of the research and the analyses of the data. Another consideration is ownership of the images: Are the images photographed-observed and described or taken away from their creators? Are the images anonymous or attributed? The answers to these questions can have legal and financial connotations (Malchiodi & Riley, 1996). All of these considerations exist in verbal settings but become more pronounced in using visual data.

B. The Observation of Creating or Choosing Images as Data

Silverman (2000) argues that research must access not only what people do but also what people say. Image making brings here-and-now action into the research situation. The action, in and of itself, is analogous to other actions: how people share colors, pages, and resources; how they handle frustration or difficulty; how they prioritize what to put on or leave off the page; and what to relate to on the page.

Mason (2002) claims that the process of creating the image already becomes a type of interpretation of the image, or part of the data. He describes how research participants agonize over the process of where to put each family member when drawing a genogram or family diagram; this is an important component of the data, which is not apparent within the finished image or genogram. The process of creation can be videotaped or observed. For example, Lallush (2012) walked around with the young girls from the slum as they photographed their neighborhood. She recorded the dilemmas that the girls verbalized of what to photograph and what to ignore: Their omissions pointed to important areas of the data. This process of inclusion or elimination can be explained by the researcher or by the participants in terms of what they experienced when creating or observing an image.

The dynamic of this process was shown in the central case study in one Bedouin woman's use of gold paint:

> A woman worked carefully on her silk brooch, embellishing it with hand paint. Yet, while she was painting her artwork, she constantly

glanced at the bottle of gold paint that was offered as an additional decoration to be used sparingly. Finally she reached over and took the bottle of expensive paint, looking around at the others, who did not notice. She began dabbing it onto her brooch design, putting on more and more.

Baron and Kacen (2012) created a research method in which participants observed a video of themselves making objects out of clay. The participants tried to identify the ways that they coped with the new experience of working with clay and to connect this to their more general coping styles (Bar-On& Kacen, 2010).

C. Explaining an Image

Ready-made or created images can be used as a method to trigger a discussion that initiates new perspectives and terms or to indirectly touch upon emotional, painful, or socially taboo subjects, as shown in the earlier chapter.

We saw in the Bedouin case study that the image becomes a trigger for a focus-group type of exploration of an issue (see chapters 3 and 4) (Benson, 1987). Each image provides an additional interpretation of the group experience (Skaif & Huet, 1998). This process allows variations of the same issue to be discussed among a group of people. For example, in the Bedouin case study, variations on the subject of houses elicited different information from different women, such as comments that houses are difficult to acquire or afford or that living in a house is confining (see chapters 3 and 4). This information can challenge existing stereotypes of how a particular group understands the issue.

Alternatively, the researcher and participant can discuss the image and infer meanings, such as in an interview. Schaverien's (1999) analogy of two people (the artist and the observer of the art) gazing together at the image as into a lighted window and both seeing new things within the room is an apt description of this dynamic.

D. Analyses of Images by Researcher

In contrast to the above, the image can be understood by the researcher or according to a metatheory, without regard to the artist's understanding of the image. Rose (1988) uses the term *visualizations* to describe how different cultures and discourses "visualize" different things in the same picture. Rose outlines the following three predominant discourses: pure content analyses, psychoanalytical analyses, and discourse analyses.

Pure content analysis is focused on noting the compositional content of the image and the aesthetic strategies used. The image is analyzed as a discrete element that is separate from a specific social context. This method is used in the analysis of fine art (Lowenfield, 1987; Mullen, 2003; Rose, 2001).

Psychological analysis views art as having regressive and unconscious elements connected to fantasy and desire, which are expressions of the unconscious mind. Images are often used to evaluate or diagnose psychological functioning, such as levels of trauma, possible sexual abuse, and psychiatric illnesses. For example, sharp, shaded, or encapsulated shapes that are apparent in the composition can be interpreted as manifestations of stress, although they may be hidden in the content level of the image (Nuttman-Shwartz, Huss, & Altman, 2010; Silver, 2001; Wilson, 2001).

The third perspective, discourse analysis, claims that the art expresses a discourse or knowledge about the world, expressing different power structures. The aim here is not to penetrate into the meaning of the art, but to understand the discourses that it represents.

Betinsky (1995) points to a phenomenological understanding of images, which assumes that the art's meaning is created through the subjective gaze of the viewer who anchors the meaning of the picture into his or her existing knowledge and cultural contexts. This understanding is widely used within art therapy (Eisner, 1997; Pink, 2001).

Another form of analysis compares composition and content. In other words, images can be analyzed according to the features that construct their shape, color, contours, and overall compositional organization or according to the semantic content and emotional meaning attached to the image. Often, the analysis of images is based on both composition and content and on a comparison between the two, as we saw in the gaps between verbal and visual information in the social workers' images of extreme poverty. This is similar to how verbal qualitative research addresses both the form and content of a text (Pink & Kurti, 2004).

This book claims that different perspectives can be combined, such as the phenomenological and the social, as in the example of the Bedouin women's case study. As previously stated, images always create more gaps in an analysis than the written word and thus can be analyzed simultaneously from different perspectives (Denzin & Lincoln, 1988; Huss, 2009b; Pink & Kurti, 2004; Rose, 1988). The social analysis offered in this book points to the importance of combining all of the above visualizations of the image so as to better understand an image from a personal as well as a social perspective. For example, in the case study of the Bedouin women, they were the primary analyzers of their images, and the second analysis was that of the researcher, who relocated the phenomenological interpretations into the social context of marginalized, third-world women struggling with a traditional culture in transition.

An example of using a multiple prism of analyses is an analysis of Joseph and His Coat of Many Colors (based on the story from the Bible [Genesis, 37:3]; Huss, 2009b). Joseph is 1 of 12 brothers. As one of Jacob's younger sons, his father spent more time with Joseph than he did with Joseph's older brothers. Jacob was so fond of Joseph that he had a special robe made for his son, a very beautiful robe made of every imaginable color. Joseph's brothers, jealous of the attention showered on him by their father, hated Joseph, especially when they saw the beautiful coat. At 17 years of age, Joseph began to have dreams that seemed to indicate that he was destined for greatness. From a dynamic visualization perspective, Joseph's suffering as a brother rejected by his brothers and thrown into a pit could be understood as stemming from his early childhood experiences, particularly the death of his mother at a young age. The colored coat could be understood as a transitional object, a metaphor for his narcissistic compensation. From a developmental perspective, Joseph's coat could be understood as a metaphor for a young man trying to define his specific "colors" in the context of his childhood and present relationships. From a social perspective, the roles of multiple mothers and the one brother who was chosen to assume the father role must be understood as the accepted frame for a collective family, which includes power struggles and competition over who will lead the family. The coat is a cultural way of visually signifying dominance. These different prisms, when used simultaneously, enable a multiple and tentative analytical prism that defines the role of the images within the research, as will be described below.

E. Position of Images within Research

Above, methodological implications of the definitions of an image, its process, and its analyses were discussed. The final decision, about where to locate the images within the research, is based on the above decisions. All of the above considerations will define how the images are integrated into the research. In other words, how the image is defined and limited, the process of constructing or observing it, and the theory used to interpret it will determine whether the image is used within the research as data, subject, or product of the research. Each of these different positions will now be outlined (Huss, 2012).

In the Bedouin women's case study, the images were the method of research; they created a type of laboratory for understanding the experience of the impoverished women. The rationale for using images as a method was to help initiate a discussion with women who would not ordinarily disclose their experience to strangers or power holders. The use of images as the research method can focus equally on the product, the process of its creation, and the reactions to the product as potential areas of data. The process of observing image making can be used as a field for observing what people do, rather than what they say; for example, how couples organize themselves on a page to create a picture together.

Conversely, reactions to an image that has been created can be used as a trigger for a different type of dialogue, such as the emotional versus cognitive understandings of an image as in the examples of the social work students who espoused systemic theories, but who displayed emotive reactions to poor people in their images such as in Figure 5.

When using images as method, then the effectiveness of the image is not defined by the parameters of fine art, such as aesthetic innovation and quality, but rather by the usefulness of the image in eliciting a hard-to-reach type of data (Eisner, 1997; Mullen, 2003). The situation of creating an image is analogized to other situations in life;

The advantage of utilizing images as a method for research is that it enables the researcher to address issues that are difficult for research participants to directly talk about due to cultural norms, issues of pain, limitations in language, health problems, or because unconscious or taboo layers of the subject are not easily accessed verbally (Andsell & Pavlicevic, 2001; Betinsky, 1995; Emerson & Smith, 2000; Huss, 2012; Pink, 2001; Waller, 1993).

Another way of using images is as visual components found alongside verbal data. This data is an additional source of information, which sometimes tells a story different from that of the verbal contents; for example, the difference between how a Bedouin woman looks and how she draws her version of the ideal woman. Another example is the doodles in the margins of the diaries of young women on a gap year in India as described by Hirshen (2012). The doodles described the young girls' hardships, while their verbal narratives in the diary focused on the heroic elements.

Additional data enable the researcher to interpret the participants' experience from new directions and to identify alternative or even opposing narratives that create a multifaceted conception of identity, as described in relation to the Bedouin women This, in turn, may enable more empathy toward the research participants that are from extreme or different situations, because they are then understood as complex individuals, defying a simple categorization. For example, as described by Ben-Ezer (2012), in relation to the extremist group's wall drawings:

> I understood that beyond the extremist political views, and the—to my mind—violent behavior of these settlers in the territories, they hold an image of spiritual redemption that colors everything for them ... when you get that, you feel more empathy even if you hate their politics.

The analysis of visual data alongside verbal data repudiates the perception that images are a separate mode of research that should be analyzed differently. Further, the use of additional data to breakdown a single definition of a participant (e.g., as being in mourning, as well as being elderly) enables the expression of multiple facets of personality and the reduction of stigmatization (Bowler, 1997; Brington & Lykes, 1996; Foster, 2007; Simmons & Hicks, 2006; Wang & Burris 1994). Indeed, the demystification of images can be understood as a way for researchers to break the dichotomy between visual and verbal ways of experiencing the world. By utilizing images within predominantly verbal disciplines, researchers can challenge verbal clichés and deepen or shift understandings of their research population (Devi, 1984; Eisner, 1997; Harrington, 2004; Huss, 2008; Sclater, 2003).

As Hirshen (2012) stated about the doodles in her diaries: "I learnt not to be scared of the doodles, they didn't demand secret knowledge about art, and they could be analyzed like words in narrative theory, according to style and content" (p. 60).

A common place for images within art history or visual research is as the subject of the research, then they can include, as in art history, analyzing a famous work of art, a community art project, or a specific artist's development of a specific image. The images can be analyzed according to different theories (Rose, 1988). The use of an image as a subject of research demands choosing an analytical prism that can be based in the aesthetic or content levels of the image. In other words, it can be a visual or a social prism. Artists claim that one cannot reduce images to a social theory, while social researchers often claim that images are only relevant to social research as a trigger for understanding people or culture (Barone, 2003; McNiff, 1995). This dichotomy can be broken by combining both directions.

Finally, images can be understood as the end product of the research. The creation of the image itself can be defined as the research method, data, subject, and end product of the research, such as an exhibition or film. Images as communicative elements with others become the central analytical axis as well as the culmination of the research project. For example, Tsederboim (2012) created an exhibition of self-portraits that simultaneously used the analytical axis of process and the end product as the culmination of that process. This direction challenges verbal research and raises questions about how to measure the quality of this image-based research product: Is it measured according to research values, such as validity, trustworthiness, and analytical strategy (Denzin & Lincoln, 1988; Silverman, 2000), or is it measured as a work of art, according to public reception, originality, technical skill, or the inherent interest of the concept? The issue here is what criteria are used to define the quality of images as research or as practice (Harrington, 2004;

Mullen, 2003; Pink & Kurti, 2004; Shank, 2005; Simmons & Hicks, 2006; Zelizer, 2003).

To return to our example of Joseph and His Coat of Many Colors (Genesis, 37:3), the type of image, method, and analysis will locate the image of this coat within different parts of the research. For example, the colorful coat could involve additional data that struck the interviewer while interviewing Joseph; alternatively, the image could be a method to reveal the roles of Joseph's family members, for example by asking everyone in the family to draw a symbolic coat for each member of the family. As subject, Joseph's coat of many colors could be understood through different theoretical prisms; for example, through psychological theories, such as Joseph's narcissistic compensation for his mother's death at his younger brother's birth; from a humanistic stand, such as how the different colors symbolize different aspects of Joseph's personality; or from a systemic and cultural stand, such as a social symbol of dominant status within the family and tribal system (Huss, 2009b). The image of the coat could also be analyzed in terms of its visual renderings over the ages. Finally, the coat itself can become the end product of the research, as a work of art, drama, poem, or dance, or as an actual woven coat.

To summarize, the methodological considerations outlined in this chapter aim to show how considerations of image definition and of the processes of creation, understanding, and interpretation define the role of images within the predominantly verbal character of research. Each of these decisions will impact the data in the same way that similar decisions on the verbal method and analytical prism impact the final outcome. From this socially contextualized perspective, images are not pure content that illustrate, compete with, or transcend words, as is sometimes romantically implied in arts-based research; they are not psychological X rays of unconscious desires or blueprints of social situations. Rather, they are all of these things at once; complex social constructs that, like words, need to be understood within the social construct of the research as a whole.

7 Art Therapy
The Missing Social Theory of Art Therapy

In the previous chapter, the creation and interpretation of images was shown to be an inherently transformative or dynamic process also within research contexts, and this becomes even more relevant when using images in therapy. However, the claim of this chapter is that the transformative quality of images should be understood as being constructed by and reacting to a specific social context rather than as a decontextualized interpsychic process. The socially and culturally constructed aesthetic mechanisms of rendering images will impact the transformation of the images and thus their meaning, and they will define what is a problem and what is a solution within a specific context.

Throughout my years of training art therapists and social workers, I have been struck with how art therapists can discern the nuances of their clients' subjective emotions in great detail, both in art and in words. However, these same art therapists will recoil in shock if I ask a question regarding social context, such as the impact of the client's salary on the emotion being portrayed. Conversely, when teaching social workers, I notice that they immediately situate problems within social contexts but consider exploring and disclosing subjective emotions as a very "dangerous" issue. Both art therapists and social workers miss out on the whole picture, which is the combination of these perspectives, both phenomenological and social (Huss, 2009b).

A social perspective remains marginal within art therapy theory, which is informed by universal psychological and humanistic theories, rather than by social critical theories. The image is often understood as an inherent individualized statement from within the unconscious or conscious layers of the self, decontextualized from social surroundings. The minor trend in social art therapy tends to focus on using the arts phenomenologically within intense social contexts such as disaster, rather than on developing a methodology of creating, discussing, and analyzing images that include a social critical perspective as an inherent part of working with images. There is a minor branch of feminist art therapy and of arts in social action (Hogan, 1997; Levine & Levine, 2010; Spaniol & Bluebird, 2002), but these are based more on

74 *Using Images from a Socially Contextualized Perspective*

transposing the above dynamic or humanistic theories onto social contexts, rather than on creating a methodology of using and analyzing art from within a social perspective.

Many art therapy clients in the public sphere, such as schools, community centers, and institutions, involve marginalized and non-Western social groups. These clients are often dealing with immigration, poverty, and other social problems (Huss, 2012); thus a social method of art therapy would be particularly relevant for them. This relative marginalization of social theories within art therapy, as compared to, say, arts-based research, visual culture, and visual anthropology as described in the former chapter, could be because, historically, art therapy was a dynamic intervention. It started with interpretations that focused on the triangular, dynamically constructed relationship between the art, the client, and the therapist. The founding art therapists were psychoanalysts, who understood images as a means of accessing the individual or collective unconscious (Rubin, 2001). The creative activity occurring between the art therapist and the client was also considered a reflection of the transitional space between mother and child, as expressed in Winnicott's theories, which defined art making as projection and sublimation—and thus positive defenses (Nuremberg, 1966; Kramer, 1971; Rubin, 2001; Schaverien, 1999; Winnicott, 1958).

Following this psychoanalytical approach, a humanistic shift occurred within art therapy theory that focused on the phenomenological understanding of the creative process, such as image making, or on art making as a therapeutic activity in itself that occurred between the artist and his image. The client became the central interpreter and initiator of images. The therapist was seen as a nonjudgmental and enabling supporter of this process, which led to self-fulfillment or to self-actualization (Betinsky, 1995; Rogers, 1993; Silverstone, 1993). This created a shift to the view of art as healing, rather than art as adjunct to the relationship with the therapist (Allen, 1993; McNiff, 1995; Moon, 2008). Cognitive behavioral therapy also utilizes images as a way to concretize solutions through guided imagery and through visualization, which are also conceived of as universal and neurological components (Lang & Bradley, 2010; Rosal, 2001).

This disconnects art therapy from the many directions in the social sciences, such as community art, photo voice, and visual anthropology that have started using images to transform society. An explanation for this gap is that art therapy has been historically focused on becoming accepted as a "psychology" and has not developed in parallel with these innovative directions in using images (Johnson, 1999; Rubin, 2001). This chapter aims to suggest a method for incorporating critical theories into art therapy practice as an additional prism to add to the existing dynamic and humanistic orientations. Indeed, images, as the meeting point between the personal and the social, are an excellent place to concretize the connection between subjective and objective experience and are, thus, particularly suitable for social critical perspectives in art therapy. When social context is integrated as an internal rather than an external organizational prism for understanding the definition process, construction, and interpretation of images, then the images reveal social problems and also socially contextualized solutions to problems and how people cope. This information is situated within a personal interpretation of social reality and becomes manifest in the image (Huss, 2010a, b, c, d). The following section will elaborate on this position with examples and point to the shifts that it demands within art therapy theory.

A. The Aesthetics of Defining a Problem and Solution from a Cultural Perspective

All types of cultures maintain themselves through common belief systems that are often organized around a set of symbols that represent those beliefs. These symbols are transmitted and also adjusted, from generation to generation. Campbell (1999) describes how lived experiences become meaningful and gain coherence as narratives when they are described or reflected back through symbolic productions. Symbols within the context of a specific culture can help to heal and fortify the individual by reconnecting her or him to the base values of the society that are manifested in the symbols (Devi, 1984; Edwards, 2001; Wolfgang, 2006), defined as a means to address the specific needs of people in specific times that are exchanged for new symbols at other times. Examples of this (Malchiody & Riley, 1997) point to the use of peer group symbols by adolescents as a strategy used to create individuation from adults in Western society. Jung (1974) describes the use of the cross as a fortifying symbol for Christian believers. Kiligman et al. (2000) point to the use of graffiti in Israel after the assassination of Prime Minister Rabin as collective symbol making that helped the country overcome its shock and trauma. The peace symbol was constantly repeated.

The aesthetic organization of images reflects a culture's values and the definitions of a problem and of a solution within that culture; For example, in relation to the case study of the Bedouin women, we saw that from a psychological perspective, a traditional worldview helps to pull the person upward into a collective spiritual and sublimated existence that, prevents regression into primary and individualized satisfactions. This worldview, when lacking, becomes the individual's "problem." Thus, an emotional problem could be defined as insufficent spiritual or moral strength to take part in the overall fabric of society (Al-Krenawi, 2000; Allen, 1988; Cole, 1996; Irving 1997). Patterns are repeated, rotated, and varied in the context of harmony and order, with all of the parts fitting into the whole. This aesthetic reflects the values of the traditional Bedouin culture, which understands the individual

76 *Using Images from a Socially Contextualized Perspective*

as part of a complex, harmonious, and regulated whole (Allen, 1988, 1993; Fugel, 2002; Irving, 1997; Naasr, 2002). On this level, the arts of embroidery, weaving, and calligraphy become therapeutic as the women "weave" the values that protect the individual within the context of a collective culture, mirroring this worldview in its repetitive harmonious and ordered designs.

Compared to this, within Western culture, stress is placed on the individual and her or his path toward finding a unique way in the world, which is expressed by and embodied in personal images (Allen, 1993; Moon, 2008; Ryne, 1991). This aesthetic is also reflected in the dominant aesthetic language of art therapy, which seeks individual self-expression and self-interpretation and encourages originality, focus on process, and interpretation over product (Moon, 2001). From the perspective of Western art therapy, embroidery can be understood as a repetitive and "nonexpressive" art form, or, at best, a calming activity, rather than a type of art therapy in itself. Because Western culture and thus its aesthetics are the dominant base for art therapy, it is often understood as a universal language that informs diagnostic tests. This creates a danger that the Western conception of image making and of cultural solutions may be imposed on clients for whom it is not culturally compatible (Hogan, 1997). However, a statistically significant percentage of omissions of body parts, encapsulations, and distractions, such as butterflies and flying birds, in pictures made by children, together with overall poor compositional integration, heavy shading, asymmetry, slanting figures, and writing within a picture are considered signifiers of sexual abuse or extreme stress in children, regardless of culture (Burns, 1987; Furth, 1998; Silver, 2001; Wilson, 2001).

From this diagnostic perspective, for example, the following case study renders a reading that is different from a culturally contextualized understanding. In the following research example, sets of drawings by Bedouin children in recognized and unrecognized villages were compared (Alheiger-Taz, 2010; see Figure 6).

A common use of images in research is as a diagnostic tool to understand children's cognitive and emotional development. However, this universal use of images also ignores cultural contexts. The children from the unrecognized and poorer traditional settlements were, not surprisingly, found to be at a lower cognitive and emotional developmental level, as compared to the township children, who drew realistic houses and trees. However, the content, as well as the aesthetic organization of the images, also shows the different conceptions of the children (see Figure 6). For example, the village children drew the traditional carpet that sits in the middle of the tent and used its colors as a background for the drawings (Figure 6, Image 3), showing traditional values and defining this carpet as an emotional center of the family (Tal, 1995). These children drew small houses with fewer details, which clustered together, thus defining "home" collectively (Figure 6, Image 2). Thus, in Image 2 we see a different conception of what is defined as a home (e.g., a tribe, compared to a house). Compared to this, the children who lived in the town house drew large and detailed houses, pointing to a higher developmental level according to diagnostic tests. However, within the social context, if a group of small homes is defined as a home, then while each individual house does not have many details (a measure of development), the group of houses can be seen together as the "details" because the group is defined as a single home. Without this cultural context then, according to diagnostic meta-analyses of developmental level (Kellog, 2005), the children would be defined as developmentally less advanced because the social context is not understood (Gardner, 1993).

Images of nature can be defined as forms of dissociation or stereotypes that cover up original experience (Furth, 1993; Silver, 2001). However, in terms of socially contextualized analyses, these decorative compositions are the solutions to problems through reigniting harmony, a form of therapy in themselves.

The following case study from the researchers' workshops used images with impoverished Tamil villagers after the war in Sri Lanka (in conjunction with the Tag Ngo) (see Figure 13).

Villagers were offered different forms of aid, including art therapy. They stated that the most important thing for them, before even basic needs such as electricity and water, was to find help in repainting the gods in their temples that were ruined by the Tsunami and war, although they had many pressing physical needs such as water, electricity, and milk for the babies. The reconstruction of their temples was a symbol of protection and healing, as well as of social action, joint construction, and coherence after the trauma of war and, as such, was a form of art therapy. Although art therapists do not have the skill to build and to repaint the temples, they have painting skills and can learn from the villagers and define or translate this need as therapeutic to power holders. They can also incorporate work with images of the different gods to strengthen and to protect within the individual therapy space as well.

In Figure 13, Image 2, we also see images in Sri Lanka used to convey didactic messages to people who don't read. After the traumatic war and tsunami, local artists entered impoverished areas and with the villagers created large murals reminding villages to be cautious of the existence of land mines and showing how to identify them; they also used images to show how to avoid stepping on live mines. The artists also created murals with the villagers that discouraged men from drinking and beating their wives in times of stress and unemployment. The village men helped to create these messages, and thus were able to internalize (Third Eye Foundation, n.d.). These moral and didactic messages are considered closer to

78 *Using Images from a Socially Contextualized Perspective*

advertising or to education in Western culture rather than being a part of therapy. However, within a culture fragmented by disaster, returning to basic values and safety behaviors can be defined as therapeutic.

The above examples have implications for the process and locations of the practice of art therapy, situating as it does art as therapy occurring on a continuing basis within different social and spiritual locations, within religious practice, within crafts and group meetings, and within the decorative process, in addition to the epistemology of Western art therapy settings such as the therapy room (Moon, 2008).

To elaborate, a sociocultural understanding of images within art therapy implies searching for socially contextualized roles, aesthetics, and interactions with images, in addition to classic Western uses. This includes a search for places where people create images that are meaningful for them and implies making a connection between art therapy and cultural contexts, rather than encapsulating the client within a psychological space disconnected from his or her use of images. Cultural uses of aesthetics and natural visual settings can be transposed, in terms of aesthetics as well as of setting, into the art therapy setting, rather than the client having to adjust to the art therapist's aesthetic and ideology. An example of such an imposition of the dominant worldview is given by Hogan (1997), who states that art therapists may claim to be culturally sensitive but actually dominate the participants by offering an art process or interpretation that is alien and strange to them.

This form of "art therapy" moves away from contextualizing the art into a closed folder and closed room. This method calls for a more complex understanding of image use in cultural and social contexts. This broad definition of what an image can be challenges art therapy paradigms that are based on Western aesthetics and social paradigms, such as the assumption that the process is more important than the product; that the product has to be original in order to be authentic and thus therapeutic; or that art has to occur within the closed space of the therapy room in order to be therapy, rather than, for example, within a temple or in a community setting.

As stated previously, this cultural stand also has implications for understanding images. In the above-mentioned images of Bedouin children from townships versus unrecognized villages (Alheiger-Taz, 2010), the differences between the two sets of drawings (urban versus rural traditional settings) can be defined according to Western developmental diagnostic parameters as the village children being less developed at the schematic stage of drawing, which is a 2-year delay in comparison to their peers in the township. The images made by the village children do not have a baseline, which signifies lack of security; their houses aren't drawn with details, pointing to less emotional stability. Indeed, unrecognized villages are often demolished by the Israeli municipality (see

Chapter 2). This gap in development as expressed in the drawings could be the overall developmental and emotional price that the village children pay for extreme poverty and political conflict. However, from a cultural social perspective, this gap could also be explained not only as lack of emotional security and cognitive development, but also as a different set of recourses or resilience that focuses on collective symbols. Arabic art tends to focus on symbolism, metaphor, and decorative elements (Allen, 1988; Irving, 1997; Kroup, 1995). Compared to this, Western art aesthetics tend to focus on realism (Gardner, 1993; Lowenfeld, 1987). This can explain why the children brought up more traditionally in the unrecognized villages, with less exposure to Western culture, are more concerned with decorative, metaphoric, and nonrealistic elements in their art (Mason, 2002; Malchiodi, 1998). From this perspective, transposing the colors of the carpet (which symbolize family unity) to the whole picture is not only an indication of lack of security and realism, but can also be understood as expressing a recourse, the strength of the family ties for this child. These drawings can be understood as describing a coherent social network that enhances the children's resilience against the lack of educational recourses and the unstable political situation that they live within (Derk, 2002; Kaplan, Matar, Kamin, Sadan, & Cohen, 2005; Laor et al., 2006). This perspective is a reading of aesthetic language, not only as manifestations of defense and stress, from a universal or western perspective, but also as manifestations of cultural resilience such as those advocated by Hoffball (2001). This resilience can only be seen or understood in relation to specific cultural location.

B. Hybrid Perspective of Images within Art Therapy

Culture is a composite and evolving element constantly reinterpreted and reintegrated by those within the culture: Houses, for example, were shown to afford protection, but also to create confinement; men were shown to deny women entry into Western culture, but also failed to protect them as they had in traditional culture. We saw how the Bedouin women from a position of poverty could not creatively integrate different discourses (Mills, 1997); and we saw that the women needed the integrative space of the image so as to define a problem and a solution within a fragmented social context. When cultural discourses are oppositional or fragmented, then, as we saw with the Bedouin women, one does not know what to wish for (Huss, 2009a,b):

> They have no narrative structure with which to make sense of their lives. They are caught at the conjunction of several opposing discourses ... [that] result in texts that are far from cohesive and which are fractured by these disjunctions. (Mills, 1997, p. 100)

However, creativity also encourages new integrations and perspectives; Smith (2002) states that conflicts between different discourses sometimes leave spaces for the individual to renegotiate power and weakness within the constraints of her life (see Figure 3, Image 9). This was apparent in the images of the above Bedouin woman who, like the other women, created new integrations and solutions to her problems by combining the two cultures within her image—such as new messages in décorative traditional aesthetics (see Figure 3, Image 9).

This process points to the healing and integrating elements of creating new cultural forms that integrate rather than split social reality. Berry (1990) defines cultural acculturation as successful when it manages to integrate both cultures, rather than to reject the original or the new culture. The ability of images to integrate different and even conflicting cultural and social narratives becomes a type of gestalt technique that creates a more harmonious and thus enabling social narrative. In the case study of the Bedouin women, for example, we saw that the women created a new discourse that integrated the Western and traditional aesthetics of the two cultures between which they are caught (Berry, 1990; Campbell, 1999; Hermans & Kempen, 1998; Mills, 1997). They learned new Western-style craft making, such as silkscreen printing, to which they added traditional embroidery, they created calligraphies of modern contexts, and they draw new versions of symbols from nature to tell their story and express their loneliness.

These cultural splits become internalized as inner psychological reality. For example, we saw in an earlier chapter how the young girls who photographed their slum neighborhood both hated the trash that permeates it and yet also "trashed" the neighborhood themselves. The social work students cannot integrate what they are taught and what they experience. The Bedouin women in the central case study struggled to decide if they were strong or weak, traditional or modern. Mapping out and then integrating these dual or fragmented social realities into a coherent image becomes a therapeutic objective of social-oriented art therapy. Indeed, the combination of these different narratives on a single page already serves to create a dialogue and integration between them (Huss, 2010c; Rhyne, 1991)

While marginalized groups cannot find their inherent voice in relation to a fragmented reality, for more powerful groups, cultural and social context are often invisible, and it becomes part of the therapeutic job to connect personal problems to cultural constructs that may create them.

This is exemplified in another example from the above-described visual genograms, drawn by social work students, then one participant drew her family as a type of cloud that wandered over Europe, due to the Holocaust. The experience of escaping from the Holocaust was a taboo subject in the family, due to its levels of trauma, and was depicted as the blue, "frozen" color. The participant described wandering across the globe, from Poland to Europe to Australia. This wandering created a deep sense of rootlessness in the participant that could not be discussed within the family, which created a feeling of loneliness. An understanding of this historical and geographical reality as depicted in the creative genogram enables us to understand and to forgive the disengaged family and internal family dynamics that became the participant's personal problem passed on from generation to generation. This was conveyed visually through a wondering cloud metaphor within which the many family divorces and lack of contact became understood.

To summarize this point, a social perspective demands that art therapists consider how the client negotiates the different (global and specific) cultural contexts in terms of experiencing splits and in terms of defining problems and solutions, and creating new integrations in the aesthetics and symbols of this image. How can a coherent reality be created in a split social context? This cannot be learned only from books or anthropological observation, but rather from the client him- or herself, who may combine different and even opposing cultural discourses in a way that is understood by and is meaningful to the individual. Within an art therapy interaction with members from marginalized groups, the art therapist is the representative of the dominant culture. This helps art therapy to avoid becoming another form of hegemonic control. As stated by Highwater (1995):

> The dominant society is rarely given the opportunity to know the world as others know it; therefore, they come to believe there is only one world, one reality, one truth, the one they personally know. (Highwater, 1995, in Goldberger & Veroff, 1995, p. 205)

At the same time, the issue is complex because due to globalization Western and traditional cultural aesthetics are more widely understood, and the client can learn the aesthetic language of Western art therapy. Indeed, this may be the only place that the individual can learn the aesthetic and cultural definitions of problems and solutions in the dominant global culture if he or she cannot afford a formal education. If it is recognized that the art therapist is teaching a specific aesthetic language rather than engaging in a universal language, then this can help the client understand Western or global culture. This was exemplified by the Bedouin women who wanted to learn Western crafts and to include images as self-expression within their groups in the central case study.

On the one hand, the most basic form of analysis that is client-centered is a phenomenological perspective based on the client's own explanation and self-integration of different cultural constructs. This type of analysis is demonstrated by Avnet's (2003) statement that art, if used as a way to accept multiple elements of identity, rather than to define or interpret identity, is a way of decolonizing third-world women. She states, "Our clients will be better served if we suspend our clinical judgments and open ourselves to experiences portrayed through art, however impoverished or unique" (Avnet, 1993, quoted in Hogan, 1997, p. 186). However, the claim of this book is that a phenomenological stand that focuses on individualistic experience, out of a humanistic paradigm, is not enough to understand this experience within its social context. In addition, a cultural stand that implies a search for culturally contextualized analytical prisms for understanding, interpreting, and bracketing the client's image construction means bracketing the subjective and relocating it within a social context, and vice versa. For example, the Bedouin women's images of houses reveal the deep insecurity of poverty, rather than an "impoverished self" that a Western diagnostic analysis of their house drawings would suggest.

Clients from marginalized groups often have intense and immediate problems in the present, as well as the burden of past losses and transitions to deal with (Robinson, 2000; Sofie & Solvig, 2000). Within this reality, phenomenological experience needs to be relocated into social reality to create a transformation of understanding for the reality. Focusing on the phenomenological can be a way to avoid a seemingly endlessly flooding and complex social reality. The art therapist needs to include additional prisms that together create a tentative stand.

If we return to the Biblical example of Joseph and his coat of many colors as an organizing metaphor for his story, then we can, from a therapeutic perspective, analyze his story as moving from the inter- to the intrapsychic, from the micro to the macro, or from the personal to the social, each initiating a different type of art therapy intervention (Huss, 2010a).

(Genesis, 37:3). Joseph, 17 years of age, is one of 12 brothers, 10 of whom are his half-brothers born to four different mothers. Joseph's own mother, Rachel, died giving birth to a younger brother. He is his father's favorite son and, consequently, his brothers' most hated sibling. His most treasured possession is a colored coat, a gift from his father.

Joseph's problem (being thrown into a pit by his brothers) can be simultaneously addressed through different theoretical prisms:

> Joseph has dreams that seem to indicate that he is destined for greatness, and he exacerbates his problematic position in the family by frequently repeating these dreams to his brothers. He arrives at art therapy feeling confused and lonely, caught up in the conflict between his father's love and his brothers' hate.
>
> Looking through the prism of dynamic therapy, the art therapist will understand the cause of Joseph's suffering as stemming from his early childhood experiences, particularly the death of his mother at a young age, resulting in his narcissistic compensation and use of

a "colorful" coat and personality to feel that he exists and is confirmed. The therapist will interpret this and bring it into Joseph's consciousness by analyzing it.

The colored coat can be understood as a transitional object, as a metaphor for his narcissistic compensation. This need will also be expressed in the transference to the therapist. Within the treatment framework, the coat is used as an additional path to access unconscious material, such as archetypes, and as an additional site for transference.

Compared to this, the humanistic art therapy prism will add the focus of Joseph's developmental challenges in the present—a young man trying to define his specific "colors" in the context of his large family and present relationships. Here, the coat can be understood as an expression of Joseph's creative and reflective individuality, and it can be used to help him integrate his identity and to find out what "color" he really is what is his authentic "self" at present, rather than being "all colors."

If we move to a systemic understanding of using images as reflecting a system between people, then the experience of Joseph's siblings' favorativsm towards him can be raised and discussed through how they feel about his fancy coat: This could be changed through asking the father to draw a coat expressing each son's special "colors."

The final perspective can be social-cultural. From this stand then roles of multiple mothers and of one brother chosen to run the familly due to age or skill are a form of social organization that is understood by the tribe: The embroiderd coat makes this choice clear and understood—similar to a uniform. (Huss, 2010a, p. 221)

This example shows that the therapist can systematically integrate theories that encompass the different ecological circles of one's life to create a rounded understanding of "Joseph's coat and problems," which enables a repertoire of art interventions or skills, each firmly based within its theoretical stand but all working synergistically together, and taking social context into account. Only Joseph himself will be able to define the most imminent and relevant analytical prism and its cultural context. The rationale for using images from this perspective is, as was shown in the research chapter, that images are flexible enough to contain opposing narratives and that they are inherently transformative. They can be utilized for different perspectives on a problem. To summarize this chapter, the ability to identify ways that images are therapeutic within a specific culture and to integrate them into art therapy was defined as an analytical prism for culturally contextualized art therapy. This process was also defined as a hybrid and phenomenological understanding of culture that in itself is the base for integrating internalized cultural splits and for transforming cultural definitions of problems and of solutions to suit the client. This forms the theoretical base for using images from a social perspective in art therapy. In the following chapter (Chapter 8), the methodological implications of this for the practice of socially oriented art therapy will be outlined.

8 Methodology of a Socially Contextualized Art Therapy

The methodological shifts in practicing art therapy through a social prism will now be outlined in terms of the different parts of the art therapy process, how a social context challenges them, including the ways in which images are defined, what is involved in creating images, and ways of analyzing them.

A. The Therapeutic Potential of Images

Dynamic theories of art therapy understand the creative process as a means to vent and sublimate intense emotions (Kramer, 1971; Nuremberg, 1966; Schaverien, 1999; Winnicott, 1958). Humanistic theories of mindfulness point to the "flow" effect of relaxed concentration and involvement in the here and now that are enabled by creative processes (Allen, 1993; McNiff, 1998; Moon, 2002; Rhyne, 1991). According to neurological approaches to image making, this flow is the simultaneous combination of physical sensory and cognitive emotional arousal, a continuing shift between mind-body and emotion, which integrates different parts of the self and helps to reset emotional equilibrium fragmented by overstimulation caused by trauma or by understimulation caused by illness or depression. This reignition sparks creativity, enabling more positive narratives to be created, and it creates a sense of physical, mental, and emotional control and relaxation, and thus, ultimately, a sense of optimism (Appleton, 2001; Conway, 2009; Hass-Cohen, 2003; Hass-Cohen & Carr, 2008; Nelson & Fivush, 2004; Sarid & Huss, 2010). This reactivation has the potential for creating new connections and pathways between the physical, emotional, and cognitive components that help to process disturbing memories held in images, and to create more enabling images and memories (Hass-Cohen & Carr, 2008; Kaye & Bleep, 1997). This dynamic situates the art process as therapeutic within a theoretical frame that is neurological rather than ideological (Allen, 1993; Hass-Cohen, 2003; Henderson, Rosen, & Mascaro, 2007; McNiff, 1989). Indeed, this therapeutic effect of image making is universal and is also activated when watching images, and it was described in a Bedouin woman's summary of the art experience: "For me, it was fun to learn something new, and especially to show my frustrations. I have a lot of frustrations as a single mother. Drawing is fun, also embroidering is fun; it's calming."

As stated in the former chapter, a social perspective broadens the definitions of what constitutes art in therapy: images within religious practice, within crafts and group meetings, and within the news media are all potentially therapeutic images for clients from different cultures. This challenges the previous method of focusing on the process rather than the product (McNiff, 1995) and challenges art therapy paradigms that are based in Western aesthetic and social aesthetics, such as a focus on originality of product as being parallel to its therapeutic value (Moon, 2000). This also challenges the assumption that art has to occur within the closed space of the therapy room in order to be therapeutic, rather than, for example, within a mosque, a temple, in a community setting, or in relation to an image in the media.

This implies that art therapists need psychological as well as anthropological and visual culture training to better understand different cultures and images within a particular culture. This can include religious or cultural settings, soap operas on TV, pop culture icons, sports heroes, and the aesthetics that go with them that may be different from those of the art therapist trained in Western fine art. As previously stated, from a neurological perspective, the process of seeing or imagining an image is identical. Projective theories also point to the ability of individuals to project different content onto the same images or to use images created by self or others as a way to search for and find meaning.

Images used in therapy can include crafts, things the client likes to see or imagine, and spaces and places that are important to him. In other words, the art therapist must identify the images that the individual engages with and uses in her own world, including traditional ceremonies and talismans (Farrelli-Hansen, 2001; Liebman, 1996).

Another example of this flow experience as well as the normalizing and destigmatizing power of art, is exemplified in a research project that involved a studio arts group for psychiatric patients living in the community (Stillerman, 2012). The process of art making demonstrates that states of mindfulness, pleasure, and self-regulation were intensified for the participants and these skills were then translated to other situations. This is shown in the following quote from this study (Stillerman, 2012):

> Miriam has to undergo an operation and is very scared; she decided that water colors calm her down a lot, and she asked her social worker to come with her to buy a set of water colors and pages to take to the operation to calm down. After the operation, she showed us the pictures and we put them on the wall.

From a social perspective, image making or engaging can be defined as an activity that enhances relaxation, communication, and pride in a product. This is a nonstigmatizing process that focuses on the whole person rather than on a definition of a problem. From a cultural perspective, society provides spaces for women's quilting, knitting, crafts, and ceramics groups, for people without special needs within the community and provide these settings. The social effect of engaging in a normal activity is especially relevant for stigmatized groups such as psychiatric patients. This effect is illustrated in the following quote:

> Julia came into the studio and looked at her picture of a camel from last week. She asked, "Did the teacher correct my drawing?" We explained that no one touched her drawing; her drawing didn't need correction. She couldn't believe she had drawn such a successful camel that didn't need "correcting," that she was ok, fine as is. (Stillerman, 2012, p. 84)

Even if the person is limited in terms of body, mind, or emotions, the image-making process engages all three of these elements to create a whole person experience; this defines the individual as comprised of elements beyond her or his disability. On a social level, this does not define success or failure as narrowly as formal areas of activity and learning do, and so it enables space to experience success and strengths.

The combination of flow and a destigmatizing "whole person" activity becomes a way of defining marginalized or special groups of people through a holistic and strengths-based theory. On this level, engaging in art is to take a social action stance. For example, a woman in the psychiatric group described this process:

> I didn't know what to draw at the beginning; I didn't connect to it; I just did colors and shapes, and then gradually it caught my interest. I started to like the colors, the shapes; it's like this process, of finding out that you are ok ... with all the problems, you are ok.

This type of dialogue demands that the art therapist cultivate the ability to create situations for engaging in art activity that are culturally acceptable and destigmatizing (Allen, 1993); in other words, to relocate art engagement back into its social context.

A case study mentioned in an earlier chapter discussed the use of art for Tamil war and disaster survivors in villages in Sri Lanka. A program utilized wounded and old people to teach traditional crafts and games to children who could not get to school. This was successful in destigmatizing all of these populations and in initiating proactive pleasurable and healing situations of "flow," as well as in restructuring symbolic forms

88 *Using Images from a Socially Contextualized Perspective*

that hold meaning. This can be considered a community type of art therapy although it is focused on crafts rather than on therapy or on art.

B. Dialogue with Pain: Mapping and Symbolizing

As described in the previous chapter on arts based research, in addition to the primary stage of sensory engagement, image making includes the stages of active decision making as to what is included in the image and the process of mapping or choosing how to represent these elements. This becomes a dialogue with the content (Kagen & Lusbrink, 1978). This explorative dialogue with the self through creating an image is described in the Bedouin women's summaries of their art experience. One woman noted:

> Drawing helps you understand what's going on inside; it lets you get out of the circle you're stuck in. It helps you think how to get out of that circle. Lots of psychologists and social workers have worked with me since my divorce, and drawing helped me more than all the talking, to think how to get out of that narrow spiral you're caught in going round and round. (A Bedouin woman from the case study)

The decisions on content or form are already therapeutic in that they provide a proactive and interpretive stand toward the content being depicted. The image-making stage includes a symbolic dialogue with the content in terms of decisions on how to depict it on the level of composition, which is the base for adjustments of meaning (Henderson et al., 2007; Sarid & Huss, 2010). This process can occur when an individual observes an image and then finds a new meaning within it or when an individual adjusts an image in his or her imagination.

> You need to continue, it's not all pink, but you need to continue, although you are angry, you have been hurt, others have hurt you, and you need to continue beyond all that; not to give up. I started drawing myself in bright pink, but then I drew over me in the color dark red—a more realistic, grounded color. (see Figure 7)

Similarly, a person observing the same image can identify different meanings in it at different times. This is demonstrated in Figure 7, which presents images of self-fulfillment of impoverished at-risk, unemployed women (Magos, 2012; see Figure 7, Image 3).

> At the beginning I wanted to paint the whole picture pink, which is happiness, because I finally got a job, and I am so happy; and then I thought, just a minute, it will take time; it's hard work. So I painted

it half purple and half pink, to remind myself that it's not going to be easy so I won't be disappointed.

Symbolizing experience enables a dialogue with that experience through compositional elements. This dialogue leads in turn to a dialogue with the social meanings of the image because the central subject versus the background can be seen as the individual or the problem, organized within the evolving gestalt of the issue and within its social context. The aim of therapeutic intervention is to transform problems or understandings of problems to create an understanding of the issue that is more enabling.

An image by definition contains a central figure, and a background or context for that figure that creates the tension within the image. Implications of this for an art therapist are to take the social prism or context of the client's life into account when looking at the image, rather than trying to decipher inner reality only through the image. This can lead to an understanding of the problem in terms of cultural context, and also create a critical dialogue with existing cultural entities.

C. Images as Revealing Socially Contextualized Solutions

Symbolic depiction that is not tied to reality can be used to show and concretize ways to potentially resolve a situation. In other words, because symbols are not reality, they can help individuals envisage or imagine solutions to problems. One woman from the group of unemployed women drew her diary and described how it was her way to cope with finding a job:

> I drew my diary because it is very important to me: It helps me keep order and most of the pages are empty, so I can see the most important things, and keep order; but I also write my feelings in my diary, and all my girlfriends have written me blessings in my diary. Opening it gives me strength when I'm feeling down. I also drew my prayer book; it gives me strength.

This becomes a blueprint for working toward a solution that emerged from the process of symbolizing the solution.

The concept of using images to envisage solutions and problems concretizes the solution. This method is a shift toward strengths-based theories, which assume that people have solutions to their problems within the social context in which they live. Focusing on a client's solutions within a given social reality, on his strengths, and on the cultural constructs that can give him strength can be understood as a form of social art therapy (Baron, 1990). This empowers the client to become the

90 *Using Images from a Socially Contextualized Perspective*

person who is able to solve his own problems in the context of his own interpretation of his social reality.

Within art therapy, the focus, as in Western society, is often on expressing and experiencing the problem, rather than focusing on self-envisaged solutions within a given social reality. Because only the client understands his social and cultural reality, only the client can envisage these solutions. When the pain is defined within a specific social reality, the solutions, in relation to that reality, can also be defined. For example, with the Bedouin women we saw that after defining their confinement and lack of mobility, the solution was to find places and times to be together: to define themselves as strong and to demand protection and rights.

D. Utilizing Social Context for a Strengths-Based Approach to Images

A socially contextualized understanding of a problem shows how people cope with a specific social reality. These coping methods are only understood in terms of a specific social and cultural aesthetic language.

In the following example we see drawings made by Israeli children who are aged 7 to 9 years, who were evacuated from localities in the Gaza Strip area. These children are from extremist religious and right-wing groups that were forced to relocate because they refused to voluntarily leave their homes in the territories (Nuttman-Shwartz, Huss, & Altman, 2010). The children's drawings and their explanations show how the children use specific cultural and political symbols such as the color orange, palm trees, and flag of Israel. The symbols provides strength, while the compositional form of the symbol reveals stress. This creates a synergetic relationship between stress and coping that can only be understood within a specific social context (Huss, Huttman-Shwartz, & Altman, 2012; see images in Figure 9). In both images, the color orange, the symbol of this group's political struggle, permeates the whole background of the image, although it is not a realistic background color. This is discrepant with the child's developmental level, which is manifested in the realistic rendering of the contents. The child explained his picture through a projective story:

> Once there was a boy called Yair and he lived with his family in the Gush. He had a strange feeling one day, when he heard they would be sent from their homes; he tried to imagine how it would feel. He asked if only their family would be sent away, and his mother explained that no, they would all go to a big demonstration soon. So we demonstrated together, all the families.

Methodology of a Socially Contextualized Art Therapy 91

We see from the narrative that this boy's parents provided the ideological frame and its political action as a solution to the problem, just as he used a symbol of this struggle, the color orange, as a background of the entire image. Other protective collective symbols are prevalent, such as an Israeli "flag-tree" that is planted and an image of the sun that is drawn as a blue Star of David.

According to diagnostic interpretations of stress (Betinsky, 1995; Burns 1987; Furth, 2003; Malchiodi, 1998; Silver, 2001), two trees with bent trunks, falling fruit, and hollows in the trees are all signals of stress. The child expresses his stress in the compositional elements, but also his resilience, in the symbols used; the images thus reveal both stress and coping (see Figure 9, Image 2).

Another example is outlined in Figure 9, Image 2, where a girl's mother is drawn at the window of her house. The mother is described as anxious and is given an orange kerchief to wear (the color that officially symbolizes the group's political struggle). The girl who drew this said of her picture while drawing it, "I am trying to draw my mother, but I can't manage to draw her, because when my mother remembers Gush Katif (the area they were relocated from) she cries. I will add an orange kerchief to give her strength." The mother, who was still in a state of high stress, was "strengthened" by her daughter using a collective symbol of a kerchief in the color orange. Once she was bolstered by the collective symbol, the child could then describe her mother's grief.

The symbolic color of orange is understood within a specific and local cultural context. Compared to this, diagnostic art therapy analyzes the gaps between content and form, or the compositional elements of art, as an expression of the pathologies of the client, under the contested assumption that art has universal and developmental elements (Burns, 1987; Furth, 1998; Silver, 2005). However, the method previously described points to the compositional elements of individuals' drawings, suggesting that when understood within a social prism, these elements express the strengths and coping power of the creator.

The ability of the client to self-define the solution, using his or her own creativity and the symbols of strength available within his or her sociocultural context, enables the creation of solutions. A solution can also be to shift away from the cultural context (Figures 1, 2, and 3).

For example, in the case study of the Bedouin women, the women indirectly demanded a right to become more Westernized on the one hand, and the right to receive traditional support rather than isolation on the other (see Figures 1, 2, 3, and 5 and Chapters 3 and 4). Similarly, the social work students described their experience as not correlating with the values that they were taught (see Figure 5).

Art therapists can understand the process of mapping and symbolizing as simultaneously expressing defenses as well as coping with and

92   *Using Images from a Socially Contextualized Perspective*

resilience to the problem portrayed. This result becomes apparent if compositional and symbolic understandings of the image are contextualized into a specific social reality; for example, the symbolism of the color orange as protective in the former example. This type of expression allows the client to use images to envisage solutions within a specific context. This technique is utilized within guided imagery, where images of disturbing experiences are adjusted to reflect a less disturbing reality or to find a solution, such as making a problem or person smaller and more distant or intensifying the color of a comforting element.

Art therapists can integrate the social context, the stress reactions, and a focus on coping in the context of a cultural reality all within the same image, by shifting perspectives from content to composition, and to reframing or adjusting the content or composition (Huss et al., 2012). This is outlined in the following description of social practitioners in a high-stress service situation, a war (Huss, Sarid, & Cwikel, 2010; see Figure 10). In the first image (Figure 10, Image 1), taken from the chapter on arts based research, a social worker describes her drawing in the following words:

> We were mostly needed to help put wounded people and people suffering from anxiety attacks into the ambulances. We were expected to talk to them and to calm them down. But it was terrifying for me to be there, to endanger my life. My mother criticized me for leaving my kids and risking my life in the middle of the war, all for a job. All in all, I feel so fragmented and stressed from these constant and opposing demands.

This provided socially contextualized "data" on her stress as outlined in the research chapter. She observed how the composition was fragmented, and her body was originally drawn without color inside, creating a sense of weakness and of being overwhelmed. The content revealed the social context, the composition revealed the stress, but also the solution, as she decided to draw all of the colors within herself, so as to ground herself, and noted that she is actually strong colorful and at the center. Once the stress had been defined as real, that she was in reality in an impossible situation, she could observe her stress reaction without blame and reframe her coping within a difficult situation as strength (see Figure 9, Image 1).

In the second example (see Figure 9, Image 2) a social worker described her stress in wartime. She stated that when bombs threatened her house in the "cast iron war" [bombings in the south of Israel, 2010], she felt the most basic sense of safety had been taken away from her; "everything around my house became black." By drawing the image, she gained a measure of control over it, and the explanation helped to redefine her stress within this context. The explanation of this stressful experience situated her problem within a high-stress social reality. She has not defined the problem as internal (i.e., overly anxious), but rather, her social reality is defined as the problem (bombs falling). This perspective becomes the "data level" of the issue and the overall solution is of course to stop the war, but at least it locates her problem within a social reality. When observing the composition she noted that she had turned her whole world into a black surround except for the house, "as if it's pressing into it, as if there is nothing except the bombs." This is apparent in the thick, black, shaded border. The content was expressed within the symbols, while the stress reaction was expressed within the compositional rendering of the content: It is important to note that instead of using an external diagnostic tool for defining stress in compositional elements, the art therapist and client together observe the composition and define the stress reactions through a phenomenological observation of the composition.

The composition also rendered her potential solutions; She stated that while her house was surrounded by black, it was still well defined and strong. She then took a blue color and added the blue background around the house (in an area that was formerly white) as an optimistic color that would ward off the "evil eye" (a familiar cultural symbol in Judaism and Islam; Huss, 2010a). She utilized a cultural symbol to strengthen the house and to reframe or soften her stress reaction (the intense black line encapsulating the house and the empty white areas) and to counteract and normalize her surroundings, because blue is also a realistic color for sky. This gave her a sense of protection and strength, as well as proportion regarding the danger she was in.

As stated, another socially contextualized way of solving the problem was to try and change the social reality that caused the problem (such as advocating for peace instead of war). This social action stance that uses images will be outlined in the following chapter.

9 Images as Group Empowerment and Action

This chapter suggests that images are excellent tools for social empowerment and action because they constitute a meeting between the personal and the social, open up fresh perspectives on an issue, and suggest different ways of thinking about and transforming the connection between personal identity and society (Devi, 1984; Freire & Macedo, 1987; Harrington, 2004; Huss, 2008; Joughin & Maples, 2004; Soja, 1989).

Spivak (1996) describe how marginalized groups can be heard not in historical, academic, and political writings that are male dominated, but in the areas of symbolic self-expression where resistance is removed from reality and thus does not threaten the central male discourse (Bowler, 1997; Brington & Lykes, 1996; Foster, 2007; Huss, 2009; Lippard, 1995; Shank, 2005; Simmons & Hicks, 2006; Spivak & Guha, 1988; Wang & Burris, 1994; Zelizer, 2003). Alternatively, Butler (2001) describes the use of art as a way to influence society by "making waves" that counteract hegemonic stands. Harrington states, "Art shows the truth of the semblance, of systems of illusions such as capitalism, and so is subversive. Because art itself participates in semblances of illusions, it highlights these qualities of taken for granted ideas" (Harrington, 2004, p. 198).

This chapter claims that, in order to use images to change social reality by influencing power holders, the issue or problem has to be organized first within the self and with a group of similar others, so as to reach a coherent socially contextualized but personal understanding of the issue before negotiating it with the power holders (Foster, 2007; Freire & Machado, 2006; Simmons & Hicks, 2006; Wang & Burris, 1994). In other words, while the chapter on using images in therapy stressed the importance of the social context, this chapter will claim that the subjective phenomenological level of image making, or personal transformation, is the first step to changing society. This connects the micro- and macrolevels of social intervention and is embodied within the image-making process, which provides personal experience of social phenomena. This method demands a use of images that is different from creating an image to impact observers, as is the case in fine art and advertising. We saw in previous chapters that the marginalized Bedouin women described in the case study used the creation and discussion of images as a space to express and reconceptualize social problems, such as cultural transition and poverty. Definitions of women as shapeless, as disconnected black clouds, as discarded ashtrays, as cows that give milk, and as trees struggling alone in the wind were all gradually exchanged for more empowering images of women as strong horses, as demanding the right to "use our hands," as suggesting solutions such as meeting together, taking a trip together, and gaining control over living spaces. This process occurred within the dual space of the individual page and the group space where the individual images were explained. One woman summarized her experience:

> I most liked the conversations: I was amazed that other women really opened up with the art and drew such personal things and told such personal stories; we realized we have the same experiences. What we most need is awareness of our rights, of what we deserve, how we can manage on so little money; the culture doesn't support single mothers. The art helped express feelings and showed us that we need to work on our rights, and then there is a place for feelings. Also, Bedouin culture doesn't encourage people to express their feelings, and so you have to be brave to express your feelings; what most helps us is talking about these problems together ... the colors, the textures. It's enriching, makes the time less boring; we didn't do this stuff as children. The older women, even more, didn't do this stuff; they had very hard lives, lighting fires, dragging water. They worked all the time; they didn't have time for fun things like this. They had pain, of course they had pain, but they would hide it. They hid their pain. They were a lot with themselves, alone. I loved drawing, I liked the group, and it was a strong group. We spoke about everything. We didn't sit in the group in silence, but everyone talked; we had the same problems. (Bedouin woman from the research)

The use of images to create a coherent group narrative within groups of marginalized people with many problems may seem like a "luxury" activity that does not answer their most basic and real needs; however, the ability to counteract isolation and to create coherent personal and social narratives that can also be used to influence power holders is an important part of empowerment.

Due to a lack of resources and a focus on basic needs, spaces for creative self-expression are often lacking for marginalized groups. Additionally, in cultural transition, as in the example of women undergoing immigration or globalization, the traditional venues for creation and social meeting often disappear; this draws individuals to spaces where people can meet and reconceptualize their experiences, then create a new enabling and coherent narrative around disturbing experiences. This level of image use claims that venues for self-expression that are culturally compatible are important ways for society to conserve as well as transform itself. In other words, marginalized women, such as the Bedouin group, need literacy skills, computer instruction, and English lessons in order to fit into the work force; however, they also need to integrate old and new knowledge bases. Further, they need spaces that help them to redefine new social avenues for self-expression and communication, which is the basis for creating meaning and a stable identity out of the rapid transitions that they are undergoing. The combination of creating images and group space to self-define images, in relation to a shared social reality, was shown to enable this integrated avenue of expression.

A. Individual Images Within the Group

The use of creativity and images is cited as an important technique to encourage learning with a critical consciousness-orientation in poor rural communities. This type of education is achieved by bringing to the fore personal interpretation and the engagement of the imagination (Ramirez & Gallardo, 2001). Thus, learners are not passively educated but must expressing themselves in their own words. Similarly, Freire and Macedo (1987) suggest that the "pedagogy of the oppressed" is an empowering form of education that uses creative methods to access the inner voices of the students, rather than just educating them from the outside in (p. 86). To elaborate, the interaction with an image begins as a dialogue with the self, as described in the former chapters. In other words, the discussion of images dominates preliminary levels of image creation, which includes pleasure, flow, action, decision making, and problem solving, as described in the art therapy chapter. As stated, image making and choice allow individuals to organize and reflect upon their personal data or experience before translating it into an image and explanation, which others also interpret and enrich with new perspectives. Image making in groups embodies this process.

The process of finding one's own words with the help of an image was apparent in the discussion of the images of the young teenage girls from the slum, who could observe and discuss the duality between trashing their neighborhood, the pain of living within a trashed area, and of being "trashers" themselves (Lallush, 2012; see Figure 4 and the discussion in Chapter 6).

> People come and sit and dirty the area, not the mothers of the small children who come to the park of course, but us; we trash it. If we

walk to our park now, you will smell the trash and see it. We look after our own houses, but we trash the public areas.

The use of images as a trigger for enriching an understanding of an issue was also apparent in the images of unemployed women who self-defined visions of self-fulfillment and who concretized and elaborated upon these visions through images that had to be explained (see Figure 7). "I want to say what I really want to say ... I drew me standing, talking behind a desk at work: to talk, to say what I want, to reach out to others. You know, I don't want to be someone who never talks, because then I can't find people to help me or who could love me."

The self-exploration and elucidation that is triggered by an image becomes a way of constructing new knowledge: Taylor, Gilligan, and Sullivan (1995) suggest that to support the strengths, intelligence, resilience, and knowledge of girls whose culture or class is marginalized by society, and whose voices have not informed psychological theories of human development, is to support political, social, educational, and economic change.

B. Images as a Group Exhibition

The individual impact of images that create variations of a theme has been described. However, the group impact of images as a joint exhibition focused on variations of similar experience needs introduction. This type of impact will become a collective statement that organizes itself around a common theme, organizing metaphor, or image. The recurrence of symbols, colors, and stories become the dominant narrative, but it allows for variations, as each picture tells a specific story. For example, the Bedouin women all drew houses, but each house raised a different aspect of having a house, such as the struggle to afford a house on a financial level, the struggle to acquire a house on a cultural level, the wish for a private space, the wish for an emotionally supportive space, problems of confinement in the house, and so forth (see Chapter 3). Images, on this level, are a natural meeting point between personal and social experience, just as the group is also a natural meeting point between personal and social experience in the here and now (Ben-Ezer, 2001; Waller, 1993). The group and the images together create a dual symbolic space, which intensifies the interpretive voice of the group and the search for a group definition of the experience of people in a similar social and cultural group. The woman, when she presented or explained her artwork within the group space, was a central actor within the group, and her image became the prop, protagonist, or duality that enriched but also complicated her monologue to the group. Images can become witnesses and cocreators of knowledge, as interpreted by the group in the context of a specific social reality. This is in opposition to interpretation by "experts" such as researchers or therapists attempting to understand images outside of their social context. On this level, working with images in a group becomes a type of group voice, or empowerment activity, so that each image is relevant to all of the group members as a type of collective exhibition (see Figures 2 and 3).

C. Images as Challenging Social Narratives

The use of images within a group of similar others can also challenge the social norms of the individual, of the group as a whole, or of the overall culture within which the group lives. For example, the previously described social work students, who drew on their emotional experience of poverty, challenged the social critical explanations of poverty that they had been taught, resulting in a confrontation between their own experience versus their formal education.

On this level, the group discussion of the images became the site for the construction of new meaning. Groups empower because individual problems are transformed into group issues, which are then related to external oppressions or circumstances, rather than to individual pathology or weakness (Jordon et al., 1991). Social empowerment, in this context, involves raising consciousness to the unjust circumstances of one's life and defining the problem as outside, rather than inside, the self. The shared social context of the group enables this process (Jordan, Kaplan, Miller, Stiver, & Surry, 1991; Mills, 1991; Saulnier, 1996; see Figure 8).

The process of social empowerment was exemplified in relation to the images of the survivors of sexual abuse (see Figure 8; Huss, Alhozayel, & Marcus, 2012). The group defined the sexual abuse as "black" and then explored different yet similar experiences of that blackness. Interestingly, only those who had experienced the abuse, and not the group leader, could interpret different facets of "blackness," such as seeing the world in black and white, experiencing the self as black, or experiencing the world as black because of the shift from a professional psychological language to that of an abstract color. This defined the women as the experts and challenged the psychological definitions of the women (see Figure 8, Image 1). Indeed, the self-created image, as a space to self-define problems and solutions, can help overcome the irony that empowerment presupposes someone bestowing power (Sadan, 1999; see Figure 8).

Similarly, the young, unemployed women, within their images, self-defined their visions of self-fulfillment as acquisition of psychological and spiritual qualities that went beyond finding a job. The aim of the group thus shifted the norms (see Figure 8). But power is not only an external event; Frankel (1985), whose work has focused on defining power in the most powerless of states, such as the Holocaust, argues that power is the inner ability to make moral choices. These women defined their values and having a job as a method to fulfill these values rather than vice versa, thus challenging stereotypes of unemployed women and concrete skill acquisition as the only thing they need.

D. Images as Indirect Challenges of Dominant Narratives

Western culture is permeated with images of women as defined by men; however, images created by participants themselves help define these areas of choice. As Jones (2003), a feminist art therapist, states:

> For women, in contrast to the linguistic tradition, art offers a means of expression which is less readily male in its vocabulary, and is therefore more readily open to and able to reference the true experience of the women. Images may speak for themselves—reducing the possibility of the artist client being spoken over. (p. 75; see Figure 2)

Indeed, challenging dominant narratives through the use of images was shown in the Bedouin women's case study. The challenge was indirect, and thus, did not endanger the individual within the group. The image spoke indirectly to others. For example, she may have discussed things within the picture that were not drawn because they were not culturally acceptable, such as ignoring one's husband (see Figure 2).

This dual interpretive level of presenting an image and then discussing it intensifies and complicates the group narrative, which can be elaborated upon but cannot be reduced to a single element. It also protects the participants from directly expressing a stand that is not accepted. Although the many different versions of related experience within the group construct a group voice or narrative, each particular interpretation of reality that is shown in a separate image can question the collective consensus. In other words, the drawings simultaneously form a group exhibition as well as an individual statement. This dynamic may be especially relevant for people from traditional cultures, where social pressure to comply with social collective values may be more intense and the individual's experience cannot be openly verbalized (Jones, 2003). This is as compared to a Western empowerment model in which empowerment is more direct (or at least, more verbally direct).

> An example of using images as indirect efforts to create social change is the Lakiya Desert Embroidery Group, which uses traditional embroidery as a way to create employment and group support for poor, widowed, or divorced women, as well as to generate financial gain through selling embroidery. The Lakiya Desert Embroidery Project of the Association for the Improvement of Women's Status aims to provide support for women experiencing social and financial stresses. The indirect goals of the center are to provide income, increase literacy, support working women, and enhance education.

100 *Using Images from a Socially Contextualized Perspective*

The women are paid for crafts they make in the center. An Arab-speaking social worker on site enables women to get advice about problems without the stigma associated with asking for assistance. It can be argued that the success of the organization is that it has transformed a traditional art form to meet new, pressing social needs. It provides a means for addressing women's problems without threatening existing social systems. Perhaps it also expresses art's subversive and energizing characteristics, in that it is creating grassroots solutions to problems, rather than relying on the external Jewish welfare services; in other words, it is turning toward culturally appropriate and nurturing forms of expression. It enables indirect confrontation with power holders by providing birth control, information on rights, and places to escape a violent husband. Proof that the organization is perceived of as subversive, despite its "cover" of embroidery, is evidenced by the many times it has been burned down by members of the Bedouin Township. However, it has always been reestablished by the women working within it. (personal communication of social worker within the Bedouin sector, name omitted for ethical reasons, Spring 2005; www.lakiya.org/lakiya-weaving/)

This process will be exemplified in the following case study of a group of women who have survived sexual abuse, which has also been described in earlier chapters (see Figure 8).

First, as described in the research and art therapy chapters, the images enabled a meeting with the pain of sexual abuse by redefining it as a color, and by concretizing the defenses against experiencing the pain. Gradually, the experience was drawn and then verbalized as "the black."

Defenses, such as dissociation through repeating shapes, or through polarization of black versus color, were made concrete within the group (see Figure 8). As stated before, only the group members could discuss the pictures, not the group leader. The group members used direct confrontation to demand shifts in the art, such as defining the hands as "attacking" (Figure 8, Image 2). This confrontation turned the women into the chief interpreters and experts, as well as therapists for each other. The issues of confronting and verbalizing the truth were thus corrected by the "group as family" in relation to the art, but also distanced by the use of images, to a level that could be tolerated. The interpretations focused on the world as wrong, rather than on the women; this interpretation is exemplified in relation to the image of the hands.

The artist defined her image: "a little girl, the hands reaching out to the girl were trying to help her." Janna confronted her, pointing out that "the hands are not helping, they could also be understood as attacking ... the hands are attacking and no one is helping...."

Lea pointed out that the red spot on the skirt of the woman in the picture is similar to blood.

The ambivalence over the hands, whether they were helping or abusing, can be understood as a reflection of the ambivalence of children regarding incest because the child both loves and fears the perpetrator. The discussion in the group context enabled the hands to be defined clearly as wrong done to the girl. The abuse was confronted, named, and defined.

Another member, Ahuva, refused to draw at all, just as she refused to take up "space" in the group. Eventually, she represented herself by placing a small black dot on a tiny piece of paper, which she then turned over and covered with many other items that were on the table. She exclaimed, "There, that's me; I don't exist."

The group pointed out to Ahuva that she was right, that she was always prepared to be a "mother" to the group members, but did not take up space for her own problems. Ahuva said that she experienced talking about herself as being selfish and bad. The group confronted this behavior and insisted Ahuva draw an image of herself and tell them about her own problems as well; otherwise, they would not share their problems with her. Gradually, she turned herself into a large white space and defined the world, rather than herself, as "black."

The group process enabled Ahuva to "take up space" and become visible on the page as well as within the group. Eventually, Ahuva started giving lectures to professionals about the trauma of incest. Toward the end of the year, Ahuva, as part of her activism, suggested to the group that they create a poster advertising the rape crisis center where they worked. They decided to create a bouquet of flowers, where each flower contained part of each woman's personal artwork from the group (see Figure 8.5). Each woman brought a meaningful picture that expressed a moment of change for her. Each of these experiences was designed as a petal that contained the personal meaning of the picture. This project enabled the message of the art to stay private within the group on the level of personal meaning; and it also enabled the women to influence society without compromising their privacy, as is often the case in court action, for example. Additionally, the art highlighted the women's creativity: they reframed the traumatic experience of sexual abuse as flowers, which symbolize purity and growth. This metaphor is in contrast to the message of "damaged goods" that the women often have to endure from society and their own inner judgment.

Further, the group experience is symbolized by the vase that holds the different flowers within it and provides sustenance as a group, with each flower being different as well as similar. For the women, each petal is also an intimate memory of a picture that was revealed and discussed within the group space. Thus, there are exposed as well as hidden elements to the image of flowers. Likewise, there are group elements (a bouquet and vase), as well as social activist elements all anchored within the same image. This poster has been presented at conferences and in community exhibition halls, with explanations about the group, aimed to raise awareness of sexual abuse and to legislate for more severe punishment of perpetuators (Huss et al., 2012). The use of images as indirect expressions remained the central organizing axis for all parts of this process.

This example demonstrates the first step in reintegrating flexibility and playfulness and reconnecting cognition, emotional experience, and physical sensation as central for overcoming traumatic experiences on the level of the image making. The images enabled the group to create indirect confrontation with the incest experience and also with the defenses that it created. This included turning the blame onto society rather than the self, and served as a product to enable the social awareness of the problem. Overall, the ability to simultaneously hold a complex reality in which the pain does not disappear but, rather, achieves symbolic expression, group reframing, and social action exemplifies a social use of images along the spectrum of research, therapy, empowerment, and social change.

This chapter has outlined the stages of using images within self-empowerment that were explored in this group first by self-defining content, then elaborating upon it with a group who had a similar experience, and finally conveying the information to others. This process uses images to explore the variations in similar experience and to anchor the definition and interpretation with the group rather than with the experts. This chapter has shown how the group space and the space of the individual page within the group create a site to indirectly concretize and explore the meeting between the individual and social reality, as a first step toward initiating social change.

10 Images in Conflict Negotiation with Power Holders

This chapter continues the previous chapter's approach in exploring the use of images for group voice and empowerment to communicate with others, in particular those individuals from different cultures or groups, those that one is in conflict with, or power holders. In Israel, there is an increase of community-oriented uses of images, rather than images as fine art in a gallery or images as therapy in a therapeutic context. This use includes images for empowerment, social action, community art, and conflict negotiation (Avruch, 1998; Barone, 2003; Butler, 2001; Joughin & Maples, 2004; Shank, 2005; Simmons & Hicks, 2006; Spieser & Spieser, 2007; Wang & Burris, 1994; Zelizer, 2003).

A. Images as an Indirect Negotiation of Power and Communication with Power Holders

Based on the previous chapter, once a coherent group narrative has been explored through images and a complex but clear content has emerged, then it can be conveyed to those outside of the group. As stated in earlier chapters, a symbol or a metaphor is less threatening or confrontational as a method of expression because it is indirect and thus remains a central communicative device in cultures that do not engage in direct confrontation to solve problems or in situations where it is too dangerous to directly confront power holders (Hijab, 1988; Mohanty, 2003). This type of message is well understood within advertising and other fields that use images to indirectly influence people. In the context of communication in interactions relating to inequality or conflict, the artwork creates a third "distanced" element, rather than a direct confrontation (Dockter, 1998; Huss, 2010a; Kellogg, 2005; Liebmann, 1996a,b). This type of indirect communication through the use of symbols, metaphors, and mapped out spaces was demonstrated in the Bedouin women's case study (see Chapters 3 and 4). The women's images enabled a space to be created that confronted and emulated, competed with and integrated differences in culture and power in an indirect way. With Jewish women, such as social workers and researchers, requests, wishes, and spatial concepts were used, whereas, with Bedouin males, whom the women are most dependent upon, the Bedouin women utilized symbolization, metaphor, and proverbs as the most distant and indirect forms of confrontation. They used mimicry, emulation, and humor to resist the power of Jewish women (see Figure 2). For example, within the Bedouin women's case study, the content of the images was often explained as an act of indirect resistance, as we saw in the explanation of the thin blonde woman, the male and female dolls, the planted garden, the wish to dress up, and the wish to use one's hands. Interestingly, different forms of resistance were used in relation to different power holders.

For example, Bedouin men were addressed through proverbs and metaphors, which are the most indirect (see Figure 2, Image 9). Compared to this, Israeli women were addressed through more direct statements including competition, emulation, and mimicry. For example, in the image of the woman who wants to be thin and blonde (see Figure 2, Image 13), the woman explicitly draws what she wants: to be thin and blonde. But the image is so exaggerated in its paleness and thin lines that it becomes mimicry (Robinson, 2000). This image uses mimicry of Western aesthetics to destabilize both cultures. I, as the Western-Israeli researcher, cannot react to this picture in an enabling way because I cannot offer her entry into Western culture at the level of personal appearance, such as being thin or being blonde, impossibilities for the Bedouin woman to achieve. For financial reasons, they cannot join a health club to lose weight, and, for cultural reasons, they cannot dye their hair or dress in an overtly Western fashion (compared to Bedouin men, who are allowed to wear Western clothes and live within Western culture). Thus, telling a Bedouin woman to be happy in her own cultural roots is not a solution because it is not what the woman wants. We see that no "right" reaction to this image is possible by the dominant culture: one anthropologizes the Bedouin woman, and another tries to sell her an impossible goal. At the same time, the exaggeration of the image also mimics Western culture because the caricature-like image shows that there are no limits to the level of thinness and blondeness demanded by that culture. Thus, the wish for this specific personal appearance is unattainable for all. On this level, the dominant culture is turned back onto itself and mimicked by the image (Bhabha, 1994).

This is shown in the following discussion around an image of a teddy bear, drawn by the women:

P 1: "This is a child and a teddy bear."
GL: "Tell us some more about that bear."
P 1: "The bear is very important for the child."
GL: "Why is the bear important?"
P 1: "Because the child gives all his love to the bear and then the bear can calm him down."

In my field journal, I wrote the following in regards to the above interaction:

> She smiles at me, and some women laugh. They look at me, testing me. I ask them if they had bears when they were little, and they said that they didn't, but that they had just learned the theory of the transitional object in the previous lesson. They wanted to see if I agreed.

In the following example, the woman exaggerates her own culture through self-mimicry and humor:

P 1: "When my kids drive me crazy I tie them to the tent pole."
GL: [I look at her in alarm.]
P 1: "I'm only joking."

The woman who made this comment lives in a house in a township rather than in a traditional Bedouin tent. In this case, the woman exaggerates stereotypes about her own culture as another form of testing and confusing the dominant culture. This type of mimicry is also present in the exaggeration of the Western as well as Bedouin culture, as in the example of the teddy bear. Bhabha (1994) claims that exaggeration can be understood as a subversive tactic, used to express the women's strength through the exaggeration of the Western aesthetic, which forces the gaze of the dominant culture back onto itself (Bhabha, 1994).

Above, we saw how resistance was indirectly expressed by Bedouin women in relation to the Jewish group leader. In the following example, we see how women from more powerful cultures and positions, such as professional social workers, trying to resist pay cuts, also use indirect methods of resistance, as in the following example (Barkai, 2012; see Figure 12).

A group of female social workers met in order to create a strategy for striking against the privatization of social work services in Israel (Alcock, 1997). They created images to raise awareness of their huge case loads, privatization of services, and low pay. They decided to create individual postcards of themselves behind the words that they had written.

We see that the images are of smiling faces behind the pages, creating empathy rather than direct confrontation. The words are written rather than shouted. These images can also be understood as a strategy that uses a space where resistance is removed from reality and thus does not threaten the dominant discourse (Spivak & Guha, 1988). Thus, also in Western culture and among middle-class groups of women with professional power, the level gender influenced the types of indirect resistance that they utilized.

B. Images as Communicating Similarity and Difference Simultaneously within Conflicting Groups

Bhabha (1994) describes cultural gaps as the "untranslatability" of words or concepts from culture to culture, each culture having its own "final vocabularies." Thus, different cultures cannot truly understand each other; however, images as metonyms mapped into spatial relationships manifest the subtle but vital differences between seemingly universal concepts such as nature, houses, or cars, when taken out of their specific cultural contexts (Bowler, 1997; Goldberger & Veroff, 1995). For example, everyone can draw a house, which is a universal element and serves universal functions of protection, identity, and so forth. However, differences between houses as tents versus houses as apartment blocks will also manifest itself in the image. In other words, both the connecting universal elements of what is drawn, as well as the specific cultural differences, will be shown simultaneously within the images, thus enabling connection and differentiation (Cohen, 2003; Liebmann, 1996a; Zeliger, 2003). The dual interpretation of showing and telling, and the dual levels of emotional and cognitive information that images contain, enable one to find commonalities and differences in images. As stated, two people who are looking at the same image have already created a commonality in purpose.

This process was exemplified in the Bedouin women's case study of the difference between a shack, a large house, a tent, and an illegally built house, which were all shown in the Bedouin women's images and defined by the single word *house*. The relative size, color, and shape help to explain additional characteristics of the content. The drawing and words become double interpretations of the experience of reality, which help to make this reality more specific and clear to outsiders, as well as to insiders and to the artist herself. This, as previously stated, includes cultural as well as subjective understandings of the word *house* (i.e., a "black house" compared to a colorful house).

In other words, mapping concepts onto a page enables the relationships between these concepts, within a specific cultural context, to be made manifest. For example, in the study previously mentioned the connection between inside and outside, between men and women, is concretized and thus clarified through mapping out their relative distances from each other. This becomes a concrete manifestation of a more generalized or internal state such as the young women from the slums' experience of "trash" as both a concrete reality but also as something that is internalized and ends up defining them and their behavior (see Figure 4).

C. Images as Encouraging Empathy between Different Groups

As described in the previous chapters on art therapy (see chapters 7 and 8), images enable sensual arousal through color, shape, and texture, which encourage mechanisms of projection that enable us to connect emotionally to an image, even if we do not fully understand what was meant cognitively (Sarid & Huss, 2010). This quality can help when trying to communicate with people from a different and maybe conflicting culture, set of values, politics, or power. As Dewey states, "Art helps take down barriers, in that the use of the imagination is the ability to put oneself in another's place ... in this sense, art is moral, because empathy is the ultimate morality" (Dewey, 1934, p. 10).

Steinberg and Bar-On's (2002) added concept of a "dialogic moment" is useful here in stressing the importance of the emotional emphatic level. When observing Arab-Jewish conflict resolution groups, they noted that moments of empathy and understanding between Jewish and Arab students occurred when a specific story or personal detail was expressed using the senses, rather than when generalized ideologies are verbalized. The page brought these specific moments into focus, adding the visual, sensual elements of form, color, and texture. These elements of empathy and emotion are prerequisites for shifts in the cognitive process of statements, stands, and solutions.

Images enable a different type of space for redefining meanings and for reaching common understanding: multifaceted and dual content and emotions are combined, showing weakness and strength, compliance and resistance. These complex stories help to break down the binary understandings of strong/weak, victim/aggressor that solidify people within one stance (see Figure 5).

This was exemplified in the images of poverty created by social workers, who understood poverty through critical social work theories that define poverty as a social problem, but who experienced it through paternalistic stands that experience the poor person as helpless and weak (see Figure 5).

We can see that images create a type of "transitional space," to use Winnicott's term loosely, that enables a more flexible interaction between two conflicting emotions, cognitions, peoples, theories, power levels, or cultures because the interaction is distanced and symbolized onto an intermediate page. If the social perspective was defined as lacking in art therapy, then conversely, the phenomenological and personal or subjective perspective is what makes images particularly effective for social change and communication. The ability of images to arouse empathy and understanding was conveyed in the social workers' reactions to the Bedouin women's images.

108   *Using Images from a Socially Contextualized Perspective*

The Bedouin co-group leader (a social worker from a wealthy family) expressed how the women's art flooded her with their pain and created disorientation about how to lead the group. This was a new perspective she had not encountered in her work with the women. Thus, the art created an effective "speech act," not only among the women but also within their larger environment, in this case the Bedouin social worker. The artwork and group dialogue of this group challenged the explanations for the women's crying. In the past, this social worker believed crying was a form of manipulation by the women to try to get extra attention or assistance. The indirect element of art helped her to relate to the women through empathy, without being directly threatened by their helplessness when expressed verbally.

Art therapy literature points to the ability of art to contain, project, and work through the secondary trauma, compassion, fatigue, and pain of social practitioners (Huss, Sarid, & Cwikel, 2010). The images also contain the "viewer's" pain and confusion concerning their lack of solutions (Malchiodi & Riley, 1996). This again, makes it an effective speech act with power holders. Indeed, as stated in the first section of this book, the social worker could not assuage the overall poverty, but she understood the women's isolation and opened a clubhouse and initiated trips because she understood their experience through their images.

Another example of using images to arouse empathy and understanding in power holders is a photographic project with a group of asylum-seeking families from Darfur, who have a negative image in Israeli society. The families were given cameras, and the older children photographed their day-to-day lives, negating the unfavorable stereotypes of them as criminal elements in society. These photographs were then exhibited in their neighborhood park, first, for them and their families to see. The exhibition enabled the experience of the youth, as self-defined by them, to challenge stereotypes and to show the family values of the group. The exhibition caught the eye of an art critic, and it was moved to an influential art gallery, where it helped raised awareness, funds, and social action in breaking the negative stereotypes of asylum seekers. The group used the camera to explore and to redefine its own experience against that of the negative stereotypes, which they could also internalize. These images held universal family elements that all could identify with. These humanizing messages helped to heal the traumatized families and showed coping mechanisms and family values. At the same time, in relation to the dominant culture, the images helped to destigmatize the community and to arouse empathy and increase the wish to ameliorate the immigrants' problems.

This experience is similar to the African American writer and activist bell hooks's claim that images have the potential to become a symbolic space for agency or a way to "look back" at people (hooks, 1984). She has described how "spaces of agency exist for black people, wherein we can both interrogate the gaze of the other and also look back, and at one another, naming what we see. The gaze has been a site of resistance for colonized black people globally.... One learns to look a certain way in order to resist" (p. 208).

This description is similar to the claim in the research chapters (Chapters 6 and 7) that mapping experience into space is a way to challenge verbal hegemonic stands by concretizing experience and moving away from rigid stands, clichés, and stereotypes. The images thus become a "political" space that resists stereotypes and lack of spaces (Soja, 1989).

The meeting between a social practitioner or researcher and client is also often a meeting between different levels of power that construct the content of the images, as described in the previous examples. We saw this dynamic in the content, process, and explanation of the images by the Bedouin women. Michel Foucault (1970) argues that power is always at play and should be reflectively addressed rather than ignored or dispelled. This suggests that art is a more flexible zone than words in terms of power struggles (Dokter, 1998; Liebmann, 1996).

An institution is often a central power holder, and the arts can help to humanize unequal relationships within institutions by relating to the whole creative person, rather than the social or pathological definition of the person (Kaye & Bleep, 1997). By shifting the communication to a different paradigm, communication between people with different levels of power is enabled. Examples of this are groups of psychiatric patients and their psychiatrists who draw images of mental illness together (Spaniol & Bluebird, 2002) or of cancer patients and their doctors who draw images of cancer and the needs of cancer patients and doctors. Wang used photo-voice to pinpoint and communicate the complaints of impoverished Chinese women to their service providers (Speiser & Speiser, 2007; Wang & Burris, 1994).

D. Images within Conflict Groups and Postviolence Forgiveness

The ability of the arts to simultaneously distance and arouse empathy is particularly relevant for conflict negotiation groups. Extreme negative emotions can become sublimated and symbolized instead of acted out. Individuals are humanized rather than categorized and similarities and differences can be safely explored (Alred, Mallozzi, Matsui, & Raia, 1997).

The arts are also useful within healing or forgiveness projects after violent interactions. Traditional crafts, as reconciliation activities, represent and explain a specific culture's characteristics in a way that is nonthreatening and enables empathy and understanding. Rosenthal (1993) describes a project in which different Serbian groups were taught each other's folkdances; Cohen (2003) describes a project of Arab and Jewish women using embroidery and oral history to represent differences and similarities between their cultures. The traditional arts, as a relatively powerless or "female" zone, compared to words, enables a less threatening content level for meeting. Kalmanowitz and Lloyd (2005), in their book on art and political violence, describes the arts as a way to help reaccess cultural memory and to enhance coping and resilience. This use of traditional arts to regain coherence was defined as therapeutic for all cultures in the art therapy chapter and not only in relation to war or violence, but in relation to cultural transition and poverty, which also fragment cultural coherence (Liebmann, 1996a; Stienberg & Bar-On, 2002).

The arts are cited as relevant after traumatic events, such as war, because they help participants to regain creativity and flexibility and allow individuals to work through traumatic symptoms of dissociation, flooding, or fragmentation in the here and now, through joint activity in artwork. The images thus heal traumatic experiences and enable it to be addressed. Enhanced coping and resilience enables forgiveness and a meeting of the other. On the level of process, engaging in a joint activity enables individuals to find commonalities rather than differences.

E. Direct Confrontation with Power Holders through Images

In all of these examples, images were used to create cognitive and emotional understanding and empathy for the "other" or weaker population. However, images can also directly confront and challenge existing social narratives through destabilizing, mimicking, or confronting their messages. Again, the senses and cognitions are engaged so as to resist a social stand (see Figure 11).

An example of this process is seen in the following case study in which young Arab women who were married before the age of 17 and 17-year-old girls who were engaged to be married describe their experiences as a "before and after" narrative (see Figure 11, Image 1; Masrey, 2011); A 17-year-old engaged girl drew her engagement:

> I met him not long ago and am very in love with him. Sometimes I think it's a little early to get married, but I know he's a good man, and I feel confident with him; I feel his support, this is the baby that I want us to have. I was adopted and while I respect my adopted mother a lot, my real mother was lacking at different stages of my life.... I will give everything to my children, and especially I will let my daughters have freedom. You know, you are respected in our culture if you are a mother, especially if you have boys, but I want also to have girls.

Compared to this, a woman after marriage (Figure 11, Image 2) described her experience of early marriage as a prison:

> I drew a young girl with a covered face who is being killed. I think marriage at a young age is like killing your daughter; I will not allow my daughters to get married at a young age. You think marriage is a white dress and a party, attention; but it's a relationship, house, children, getting used to a whole new family. I was a young child; I didn't know how to make decisions, and I was irresponsible. I thought marriage would bring freedom and joy forever, but I ended up being strangled.

The married women came to a group of young women to help them decide whether to get married at a young age. Because this message was within women's groups, it could be safely discussed, but the images enabled the intensity of the women's regret over marrying young to be conveyed to the younger women through symbols and metaphors.

Butler (2001) describes the use of art as a way to influence society by "making waves" that counteract hegemonic stands. The images of this group describe such "waves" but in a culturally sanctioned setting as compared to direct art confrontations as described below.

Psychological interventions aim to help reintegrate a person into his societal norms, whereas a social action aims to change the social stand that caused the problem. Thus, direct confrontation can be an effective method of arousing the interest of the media. Aesthetic mechanisms are deliberately chosen to shock, destabilize, or confront issues. New perspectives on issues are initiated through the compositional and content elements of the image (Brington & Lykes, 1996; Harrington, 2004; Hills, 2001; Shank, 2005). This is a definition of an image that utilizes the effectiveness of a product rather than the process. This often includes the use of words, such as graffiti, that intensify the social message. The aim is convey a clear message rather than to create a multifaceted type of art. As Butler states, "artists' collective projects curve and spread around obstacles; they vibrate, and radiate new possibilities. They make a difference. Hey, make waves" (Butler, 2001, p. 15; see Figure 9).

The use of words within images as direct resistance was apparent in some of the artworks previously seen. For example, in the images of relocated children from extremist right wing groups in Israel (Figure 9), nearly all of the images included written slogans used in the community's political struggle, such as "Gush Katif is my home" or "Gush Katif forever." These slogans can be likened in their style to graffiti, which is typically a subversive message of a resistant minority, just as this group is in Israel. We have seen the gap between words and images used to create new meanings; however, arts used to influence others or to convey a strong ideology use writing as an inherent part of the content, which is interchangeable in meaning with visual symbols. This is also demonstrated in the example of the word *home* juxtaposed with a small picture of a house in the children's pictures. Similarly, from a psychological, interpretive perspective, writing is a sign of the artist lacking confidence that she or he will be understood or heard. Religious art also uses words and letters as symbols that hold mystical and powerful meanings and express a clear ideology (Burns, 1987; Furth, 1998; Jung, 1974).

11 Summary

On the level of research, this book has shown how images constitute a multifaceted activity that includes their definition, process, product, and interpretation. This complex use of images as a method in social science creates a dialectics between content and composition and between words and images. This creates a more multifaceted type of data or intervention, which challenges socially acceptable verbal assumptions and enables individuals to show oppressions and lack of spaces that are hidden behind words. However, the images also reveal strengths and resistances of individuals rather than a stand of helplessness toward a social context. In other words, issues were made visible through understanding symbols and compositions as part of, but also as a reaction to, a specific social structure.

On the level of art therapy, this book suggested that a social theory should be included within art interventions. A social problem but also stress reactions to the social context as well as ways with which this context was coped with, were shown to be synergetic and only understood within a specific cultural reality made visible through understanding symbols and compositions as part of but also as a reaction to a specific social structure. Art therapists were called on to broaden definitions of images, processes, and interpretations as a social construct rather than as a universal or personal definition, using multiple prisms of analyses of the images.

On the level of group empowerment, the dual spaces of group and page were shown to intensify and to concretize the connection between individual and social or group experience, enabling a redefinition of social norms according to the phenomenological interpretations on the individual page and creating a clear and coherent definition of needs. This definition enabled the group to redefine a processed narrative of their experience of a specific social position through constant tension and interaction between personal and group experience, which is distanced onto and concretized by images.

On the level of dialogue with power holders, resistance as expressed in images was indirect and multifaceted. This aroused empathy and understanding. Images were also shown to be effective ways to create empathy, yet distant enough to enable a meeting of the difficult experiences of others both clients and conflicted groups, and to shift stereotypes. Additionally, images were used as direct but nonverbal confrontation aimed at destabilizing existing social narratives. These three levels of individual, group, and others are demonstrated in Figure 14.

As described in the Introduction, the central case study presented here is of the impoverished Bedouin women with whom I held image-based workshops in the basements of buildings or in huts in their village. On the days we were lucky, the old fan whirled, bringing a respite from the intense heat. The room at times reverberated with lively stories about the women's drawings and emotional closeness; at other times, silence filled the room. When I suggested that we summarize the meaning of these crafts and drawing sessions, the women nodded their heads politely and thanked me, ignoring my questions.

The questions that these workshops raised and that have been the issues explored within this book are how does the joint construction and explanation of images impact our understanding of social context and our ability to transform that context?

This case study and all the additional vignettes in the book aimed to show how images can serve as an anchor and meeting space between social context and subjective experience. Images are transformative as research, therapy, empowerment, and direct social action, when used to encompass socially contextualized definitions, processes, and explanations. The images described in this book served as research data, therapy, empowerment, and a vehicle for social change, in an evolving process that includes all of these levels simultaneously. In all of the examples in the research, the images were a way to explain, react, and transform social reality from the inside out.

This book has called for a reciprocal "shift" in taking back preconceived psychological, aesthetic, cultural, and political stands and in listening to how all these elements together are used in the distanced and integrative space of an image. All of these examples point to the usefulness of images within social research and practice including education, psychology, geography, political science, and other fields that are often not aware of each other's methods and theoretical perspectives when using images.

This has been the aim of this book, to suggest a systematic, theoretical base for the inclusion of images in social science and practice that crosses over the different fields and that enriches each field. This aim demands the use of images as method in a complex way that includes examining process, product, and interpretation, as well as placement and use of images within specific social contexts. This will enable researchers to work with the synergetic connection between words and images in different ways to transform knowledge, the individual, the group, and maybe society.

Bibliography

Abu-Baker, H. (2002). Comments on otherness, equality and multi-culturalism. *Faces, 22,* 285–298. (Hebrew)

Abu-Kuider, S. (1994). Girl's school drop-out from the Bedouin educational system. *Notes on the Bedouin, 34,* 6–23.

Abu-Lughod, L. (1991). Writing against culture. In R. Fox (Ed.), *Recapturing anthropology: Working in the present* (pp. 138–161). Santa Fe, NM: School of American Research.

Abu-Lughod, L. (1993). *Writing women's worlds: Bedouin stories.* Berkeley: University of California Press.

Abu-Said, I., & Champagne, D. (Eds.). (2005). *Indigenous education and empowerment: International perspectives.* Lanham, MD: Altamira Press.

Afkhami, M. (1995). *Faith and freedom in woman's human rights in the Muslim world.* London: Taurus Press.

Al-Ataana, M. (1993). *Connection between marital status of Bedouin woman and her self-image and psychological well-being* (Master's thesis). Bar-Ilan University, Tel Aviv, Israel.

Al-Ataana, M. (2002). *Bedouin women's welfare in a time of cultural and social change* (Doctoral dissertation). Bar-Ilan University, Tel Aviv, Israel.

Alcock, P. (1997). *Understanding poverty.* London: Macmillan.

Al-Hamamdeh, M. (2004). *From the treasures of the forefathers: Bedouin meaningful tales.* Beer Sheva, Israel: The Center for Bedouin Studies and Development.

Alheiger-Taz, S. (2010). *The experience of Bedouin children living in recognized versus unrecognized villages as expressed in drawings* (Master's thesis). Ben-Gurion University, Beer Sheva, Israel.

Al-Krenawi, A. (2000). *Ethno-psychiatry among the Bedouin-Arab of the Negev.* Tel Aviv, Israel: Hakibbutz HaMeuchad.

Al-Krenawi, A., Graham, J. R., & Maoz, B. (1996). The healing significance of the Negev Bedouin dervish. *Social Sciences and Medicine, 43,* 13–21.

Allen, P. (1993). *Art is a way of knowing.* Boston, MA: Shambhala Press.

Allen, T. (1988). *Five essays on Islamic art.* Sebastopol, CA: Solipsist Press.

Allred, K. G., Mallozzi, J. S., Matsui, F., & Raia, C. P. (1997). The influence of anger and compassion on negotiation performance. *Organizational Behavior and Human Decision Processes, 70,* 175–187.

Alush, M. (2012). Meet my neighborhood: The experience of young girls living in a well-known slum through photographs. In E. Huss, L. Kacen, & E.

Hirshen (Eds.), *Creating research, researching creations* (pp. 53–67). Bialik, Israel: Ben-Gurion University Press.

Andsell, G., & Pavlicevic, M. (2001). *Beginning research in the arts therapies.* London: Jessica Kingsley.

Appleton, V. (2001). Avenues of hope: Art therapy and the resolution of trauma. *Art Therapy, 18*(1), 6–13.

Arnheim, R. (1996). *The split and the structure: Twenty-eight essays.* Berkeley: University of California Press.

Ashford, M. W., & Huet-Vaughn, Y. (1997). The impact of war on women. In B. S. Levy & V. W. Sidel (Eds.), *War and public health* (pp. 186–196). New York: Oxford University Press; Washington, DC: American Public Health Association.

Avruch, K. (1998). *Culture and conflict resolution.* Washington, DC: Institute of Peace.

Bailey, Y. (2002). The religious conception of the Bedouin. *Notes on the Bedouin, 34,* 56–81.

Barakat, H. (1993). *The Arab world, society, culture and state.* Los Angeles: University of California Press.

Barkai, N. (2012). *Using arts for resistance in social work* (Master's thesis). Ben-Gurion University, Beer Sheva, Israel.

Baron, R. A. (1990). Environmentally induced positive affect: Its impact on self-efficacy, task performance, negotiation, and conflict. *Journal of Applied Social Psychology, 20,* 368–384.

Bar-On, T., & Kacen, L. (2012). Qualitative method in arts based research. In E. Huss, L. Kacen, & E. Hirshen (Eds.), *Creating research, researching creations* (pp. 139–159). Bialik, Israel: Ben-Gurion University Publishing.

Barone, T. (2003). Challenging the educational imaginary. *Qualitative Inquiry, 9*(2), 202–218.

Bar Tzvi, S. (1986). Traditions and ancient customs of the Negev Bedouin. *Notes on the Bedouin, 17,* 27–30.

Bar Tzvi, S. (1990). *Tradition and art of the Bedouin in the Negev.* Beer Sheba, Israel: Joe Alon Center for Bedouin Culture.

Bastien, D., & Bruce, A. (1997). Identity formation in the shadow of conflict: Projective drawings by Palestinian and Israeli Arab children from the West Bank and Gaza. *Journal of Peace Research, 34*(2), 217–231.

Bell, C. E., & Robbins, S. J. (2007). Effect of art production on negative mood: A randomized, controlled trial. *Art Therapy: Journal of the American Art Association, 24*(2), 71–75.

Ben-David, T. (1981). *Change and modernization.* Jerusalem, Israel: Kaneh. (Hebrew)

Ben-Ezer, G. (2012). The collective creative space as a tool with inter-cultural work: Group work with Ethiopian immigrants. In L. Kacen & R. Lev-Wiesel (Eds.), *Group work in a multicultural society* (pp. 149–163). Tel Aviv, Israel: Cherikover. (Hebrew)

Benson, J. (1987). *Working more creatively with groups.* London: Tavistock.

Ben Zvi, T., & Lerer, Y. (2001). *Self-portrait: Palestinian women's art.* Tel Aviv, Israel: Andalus.

Berry, M. (1990). Psychology of acculturation. In J. Berman (Ed.), *Nebraska symposium on motivation, 1989: Cross-cultural perspectives* (pp. 201–234). Lincoln: University of Nebraska Press.

Betinsky, M. (1995). *What do you see? Phenomenology of therapeutic art experience.* London: Jessica Kingsley.
Bhabha, H. K. (1994). *The location of culture.* London: Routledge.
Bowler, M. (1997). Problems with interviewing: Experiences with service providers and clients. In G. Miller & R. Dingwall (Eds.), *Context and method in qualitative research* (pp. 66–77). London: Basic Books.
Brington, C., & Lykes, M. (1996). *Myths about the powerless: Contesting social inequalities.* Philadelphia, PA: Temple University Press.
Burns, R. C. (1987). *Kinetic-house-tree-person drawings (KHTP): An interpretive manual.* New York: Brunner/Mazel.
Butler, M. L. (2001). Making waves. *Women's Studies International Forum,* 4(3), 387–399.
Campbell, J. (Ed.). (1999). *Art therapy, race, and culture.* Philadelphia, PA: Jessica Kingsley.
Canclini, N. (1996). *Strategies for entering and leaving modernity.* Minneapolis: Minnesota University Press.
Chamberlayn, P., & Smith, M. (2008). *Art creativity and imagination in social work practice.* London: Routledge.
Cohen, C. (2003). Engaging with the arts to promote coexistence. In A. Chayes & M. Ninaow (Eds.), *Imagine coexistence* (pp. 267–293). San Francisco, CA: Jossey-Bass.
Cohen, M. (1999). The status of Bedouin women in Israel economic and social changes. *Maof Vemeaseh, 5,* 229–237. (Hebrew)
Cole, M. (1996). *Cultural psychology. A once and future discipline.* Boston, MA: Harvard University Press.
Collins, P. (1990). *Black feminist thought: Knowledge, consciousness, and the politics of empowerment.* Boston, MA: Unwin Hyman Press.
Conway, M. A. (2009). Episodic memories. *Neuropsychologia,* 47(11), 2305–2313.
Curl, K. (2008). Assessing stress reduction as a function of artistic creation and cognitive focus. *Art Therapy: Journal of the American Art Association,* 25(2), 164–169.
Cwikel, J. (2002). *Health and well-being of Bedouin women in the Negev.* Be'er Sheva, Israel: Center for Research in Bedouin Society and Center for Research and Promotion of Women's Health.
Dalebroux, A., Goldstein, T., & Winner, E. (2008). Short-term repair through art-making: Positive emotion is more effective than venting. *Motive Emot,* 32, 288–295.
Dallow, J. (2007). Bridging feminist art, activism, and theory. [A review of three contemporary texts]. *NWSA Journal,* 19(1), 166–174.
Denzin, N., & Lincoln, Y. (1988). *Collecting and interpreting qualitative materials.* London: Sage.
Denzin, N., & Lincoln, Y. (2000). *Handbook of qualitative research.* Thousand Oaks, CA: Sage.
De Petrillo, L., & Winner, E. (2005). Does art improve mood? A test of a key assumption underlying art therapy. *Art Therapy: Journal of the American Art Association,* 22(4), 205–212.
Devi, S. (1984). *Symbolization and creativity.* New York: International University Press.

Derk, V. (2002). Children's sense of place in northern New Mexico. *Journal of Environmental Psychology*, 22(1–2), 157–169.

Dickson, C. (2007). An evaluation study of art therapy provision in a residential addiction treatment programme (ATP). *International Journal of Art Therapy: Formerly Inscape*, 12, 1–27.

Dwairy, M. (2004). *Culturally sensitive revision of personality theories and psychotherapeutic approaches: A model of intervention for the collective client.* Paper presented at the conference on Psycho-Social Challenges of Indigenous Societies: The Bedouin Perspective, Ben-Gurion University of the Negev, Israel.

Dwivedi, K. (1997). *Enhancing parental skills: A guidebook for professionals working with parents.* New York: Wiley.

Edwards, M. (2001). Jungian art therapy. In J. Rubin (Ed.), *Approaches to art therapy* (pp. 81–94). Philadelphia, PA: Brunner-Mazel.

Eidelman, D. (2002). *The Middle East and Central Asia: An anthropological approach.* Upper Saddle River, NJ: Prentice Hall.

Eisenhardt, K. (2002). Building theories from case study research. In M. Hubberman & M. Miles (Eds.), *The qualitative researchers companion* (pp. 5–37). Thousand Oaks, CA: Sage.

Eisner, E. (1997). The promises and perils of alternative forms of data representation. *Educational Researcher*, 26(6), 4–20.

Emerson, M., & Smith, P. (2000). *Researching the visual: Images, objects, contexts, and interactions in social.* London: Sage.

Farrelli-Hansen, M. (Ed.). (2001). *Spirituality and art therapy.* London: Jessica Kingsley.

Fine, M. (1994). Working the hyphens, reinventing self and other. In N. Denzin & Y. Lincoln (Eds.), *Handbook of qualitative research* (pp. 70–82). Thousand Oaks, CA: Sage.

Foster, V. (2007). Ways of knowing and showing: Imagination and representation in feminist participatory social research. *Journal of Social Work Practice*, 21(3), 361–276.

Foucault, M. (1970). *The order of discourse: An archeology of the human sciences.* London: Tavistock Press.

Francis, M. (1985). Children's use of open space in village homes. *Children's Environments Quarterly*, 1, 36–38.

Frankel, V. (1985). *Man's search for meaning.* New York. Washington Square Press.

Freire, P., & Macedo, D. (1987). *Literacy, reading the word and the world.* London: Routledge.

Fugel, T. (2002). The language of the dress of the Negev Bedouin women. *Notes on the Bedouin*, 34, 217–223.

Furth, G. (1998). *The secret world of drawings: A Jungian approach to art therapy.* Toronto, Canada: Inter City Books.

Gardner, H. (1993). *Multiple intelligences: The theory in practice.* New York: Basic Books.

Gerson, K., & Horovits, R. (2002). Observing and interviewing. In T. May (Ed.), *Qualitative research in action* (pp. 199–224). London: Sage.

Goldberger, N., & Veroff J. (1995). *Culture and psychology reader.* New York: University Press.

Gombrich, E. H. J., & Eribon, D. (1993). *Conversations on art and science.* New York: Abrams.
Hansen F. (2001). *Living the connection. Spirituality and art therapy.* London: Jessica Kingsley.
Harrington, A. (2004). *Art and social theory: Sociological arguments in aesthetics.* London: Polity.
Harvey, J. (2002). *Perspectives on loss and trauma assaults on the self.* Thousand Oaks, CA: Sage.
Hass-Cohen, N. (2003). Art therapy mind body approaches. *Progress: Family Systems Research and Therapy, 12,* 24–38.
Hass-Cohen, N., & Carr, R. (2008). *Art therapy and clinical neuro-science.* London: Jessica Kingsley.
Henderson, P., Rosen, D., & Mascaro, N. (2007). Empirical study on the healing nature of mandalas. *Psychology of Aesthetics, Creativity, and the Arts, 1*(3), 148–154.
Hermans, J., & Kempen, J. (1998). Moving cultures: The perilous problems of cultural dichotomies in a globalizing society. *American Psychologist, 53,* 1111–1120.
Hijab, N. (1988). *Women-power: The Arab debate over women and work.* Cambridge, England: Cambridge University Press.
Hills, P. (2001). *Modern art in the USA: Issues and controversies of the 20th century.* Upper Saddle River, NJ: Prentice-Hall.
Hirshen, E. (2012) Doodles in the diaries of young women on a gap year in India. In E. Huss, L. Kacen, & E. Hirshen (Eds.), *Creating research, researching creations* (pp. 53–67). Bialik, Israel: Ben-Gurion University Press. (Hebrew)
Hocoy, D. (2002). Cultural issues in art therapy theory. *Art Therapy: Journal of the American Art Therapy Association, 19*(4), 141–146.
Hoffball, S. (2001). The influence of culture community and the nested-self in the stress process: Advancing conservation of resources theory. *Applied Psychology: An International Journal, 50,* 337–421.
Hogan, S. (1997). *Feminist approaches to art therapy.* New York: Routledge.
Holmes, E. P. (2003). *Daughters of Tunis: Women, family and networks in a Muslim city.* Seattle, WA: University of Washington Press.
hooks, b. (1984). *Feminist theory: From margin to center.* Boston: South Press.
Hubberman, M., & Miles, M. (2002). Reflections and advice. In M. Hubberman & M. Miles (Eds.), *The qualitative researchers companion* (pp. 393–399). Thousand Oaks, CA: Sage.
Hudson, F. (1960). Pictorial depth perception in African groups. *Journal of Social Psychology, 52,* 183–208.
Huss, E. (2004). To smell the wind: Using drawing in the training of Bedouin early childhood professionals by a Jewish teacher. In M. C. Powell & V. Marcow Speiser (Eds.), *The arts, education, and social change: Little signs of hope* (pp. 75–87). New York: Lang.
Huss, E. (2007). Symbolic spaces: Marginalized Bedouin women's art as self-expression. *Journal of Humanistic Psychology, 47*(3), 306–319.
Huss, E. (2008). Shifting spaces and lack of spaces: Impoverished Bedouin women's experience of cultural transition through arts-based research. *Visual Anthropology, 21*(1), 58–71.

Huss, E. (2009a). A case study of Bedouin women's art in social work: A model of social arts intervention with "traditional" women negotiating Western cultures [Special issue: Cultures in Transition]. *Social Work Education*, 28(6), 598–616.

Huss, E. (2009b). "A coat of many colors": Towards an integrative multilayered model of art therapy. *The Arts in Psychotherapy*, 36(3), 154–160.

Huss, E. (2010a). Bedouin women's embroidery as female empowerment. In C. Moon (Ed.), *Materials and media in art therapy* (pp. 215–231). London: Routledge.

Huss, E. (2010b). A social-critical reading of indigenous women's art: The use of visual data to "show" rather than "tell" of the intersection of different layers of oppression. In S. Levine & E. Levine (Eds.), *Arts and social change* (pp. 89–101). London: Jessica Kingsley.

Huss, E. (2010c). A social-critical reading of indigenous women's art: The use of visual data to "show" rather than "tell" of the intersection of different layers of oppression. In S. Levine & E. Levine (Eds.), *Arts and social change* (pp. 217–221). London: Jessica Kingsley.

Huss, E. (2010d). Qualitative critical arts-based research. In L. Kacen & M. Krumer-Nevo (Eds.), *Qualitative research in Israel* (pp. 316–332). (Hebrew)

Huss, E. (2012). What we see and what we say: Combining visual and verbal information within social work research. *British Journal of Social Work*, 1, 1–25.

Huss, E., Alhozeyel, E., & Marcus, E. (2012). Drawing in group work as an anchor for integrating the micro and macro levels of intervention within incest survivors. *Clinical Social Work*, 3, 154–160.

Huss, E., & Cwikel J. (2005). Researching creations: Applying arts-based research to Bedouin women's drawings. *International Journal of Qualitative Methods*, 4(4), 1–16.

Huss, E., & Cwikel, J. (2007). Houses, swimming pools, and thin blonde women: Arts based research through a critical lens with impoverished Bedouin women in Israel. *Qualitative Inquiry*, 13(7), 960–988.

Huss, E., & Cwikel J. (2008a). Embodied drawings as expressions of distress among impoverished single Bedouin mothers. *Archives of Women's Mental Health*, 11(2), 137–147.

Huss, E., & Cwikel J. (2008b). "It's hard to be the child of a fish and a butterfly": Creative genograms bridging objective and subjective experiences. *Arts in Psychotherapy*, 35(2), 171–180.

Huss, E., Huttman-Shwartz, O., & Altman, A. (in press). The role of collective symbols as enhancing resilience in children's art. *Arts in Psychotherapy*.

Huss, E., Kacen, L., & Hirshen, E. (2012). *Researching creations, creating research: Social arts based research*. Beer Sheva, Israel: Ben-Gurion University Press.

Huss, E., Sarid, O., & Cwikel, J. (2010). Using art as a self-regulating tool in a war situation: A model for social workers. *Health and Social Work*, 35(3), 201–211.

Irving, R. (1997). *Islamic art in context*. New York: Abrams Press.

Jayanthi, M. (2002, April). *Opening the black box: An interdisciplinary conversation on negotiating cultural realities with children*. Paper presented at Tufts University Center for Children, Massachusetts.

Johnson, D. (1999). *Essays on the creative arts therapies: Imaging the birth of a profession.* Springfield, IL: Charles C. Thomas.
Jones, A. (2003). *The feminism and visual culture reader.* London: Routledge.
Jordan, J., Kaplan, A., Miller, J., Stiver, I., & Surry, J. (1991). *Women's growth in connection. Writings from the Stone Center.* New York: Guilford Press.
Joseph, S. (1999). *Intimate selving in Arab families.* Syracuse, NY: Syracuse University Press.
Joughin, J., & Maples, S. (2004). *The new aestheticism.* Manchester, England: Manchester University Press.
Jung, C. G. (1974). *Man and his symbols.* London: Aldus Books.
Kacen, L., & Lev-Wiesel, R. (Eds.). (2002). *Group work in a multicultural society.* Tel Aviv, Israel: Cherikover.
Kagen, S., & Lusbrink, K. (1978). The expressive therapies continuum. *Art Psychotherapy, 5,* 170–181.
Kalmanowitz, D., & Lloyd, B. (2005). Art therapy and political violence. In D. Kalmanowitz & B. Lloyd (Eds.), *Art therapy and political violence: With art, without illusion* (pp. 16–34). London: Routledge.
Kaplan, C. (1997). Working with poor ethnic minority adolescents and their families: An ecosystemic approach. In E. P. Congress (Ed.), *Multicultural perspectives in working with families* (pp. 61–76). New York: Springer.
Kaplan, F. (2000). Now and future ethno-cultural issues. *Journal of the American Art Therapy Society, 19*(2), 65–79.
Kaplan, X., Matar, M. A., Kamin, R., Sadan, T., & Cohen, H. (2005). Stress-related responses after 3 years of exposure to terror in Israel: Are ideological-religious factors associated with resilience? *The Journal of Clinical Psychiatry, 66*(9), 1146–1154.
Kapri, H., Roznik, R., & Budekat, B. (2002). *Welfare services in the unrecognized settlements.* Tel Aviv, Israel: Israeli Ministry of Welfare Study Project. (Hebrew)
Karaz, A. (2005). Marriage depression and illness: Psychosomatic models in a south Asian immigrant community. *Psychology in Developing Societies, 17,* 161–180.
Kaufman, R., Huss, E., & Segal-Engelchin, D. (2011). Social work students' changing perceptions of social problems after a year of community intervention. *Social Work Education, 30*(8), 911–931.
Kaye, S., & Bleep, M. (1997). *Arts and healthcare.* London: Jessica Kingsley.
Kellogg, S. (2005). *Weaving the past: A history of Latin America's indigenous women from the pre-Hispanic period to the present.* New York: Oxford University Press.
Kisthardt, W. (1997). The strengths model of case management: Principles and helping functions. In D. Saleebey (Ed.), *The strengths perspective in social work practice* (2nd ed., pp. 97–113). White Plains, NY: Longman.
Knowles, J. G., & Cole, A. L. (2008). *Handbook of the arts in qualitative research: Perspectives, methodologies, examples, and issues.* Thousand Oaks, CA: Sage.
Kramer, E. (1971). *Art therapy with children.* New York: Schocken Books.
Kramer, E. (2000). *Art as therapy.* London: Jessica Kingsley.
Kroup, P. (1995). *Drawing by Bedouin children from the Negev in Israel.* Beer Sheva, Israel: Kaye College of Education.

Lallush, M. (2012). Young Girls images of their home as a slum. In E. Huss, L. Kacen, & E. Hirshen (Eds.), *Creating research, researching creations* (pp. 53–67). Bialik, Israel: Ben-Gurion University Press. (Hebrew)

Laor, N., Wolmer, L., Alon, M., Siev, J., Samuel, E., & Toren, P. (2006). Risk and protective factors mediating psychological symptoms and ideological commitment of adolescents facing continuous terrorism. *The Journal of Nervous and Mental Disease, 194*(4), 275–278.

Lawler, M. (2002). Narrative in social research. In T. May (Ed.), *Qualitative research in action* (pp. 242–259). London: Sage.

Lazarus, R. S., & Folkman, S. (1984). *Stress, appraisal, and coping*. New York: Springer.

Lazreg, M. (1994). *The eloquence of silence: Algerian women in question*. New York: Routledge.

Levi-Wiener, N. (2004, July). *In between two worlds: A narrative analysis of the Druze women and higher education*. Paper presented at the conference on Psycho-Social Challenges of Indigenous Societies, The Bedouin Perspective, Ben-Gurion University of the Negev.

Levine, S., & Levine E. (Eds.). (2010). *Arts and social change*. London: Jessica Kingsley.

Levy, P. (1997). *Method meets art: Arts-based research practice*. New York: Guilford.

Lewando-Hundt, G. (1976). Conflict styles between Bedouin women. *Notes on the Bedouin, 7*, 15–30.

Lewando-Hundt, G. (1978). *Women's power and settlement: The effect of settlement on the positions of Negev Bedouin women* (Doctoral dissertation). University of Edinburgh, Scotland.

Liebmann, M. (Ed.). (1996a). *Arts approaches to conflict*. London: Jessica Kingsley.

Liebmann, M. (1996b). Giving it form: Exploring conflict through art. In M. Liebmann (Ed.), *Arts approaches to conflict* (pp. 152–173). London: Jessica Kingsley.

Lindsfore-Tapper, T., & Ingham, B. (1997). *Languages of dress in the Middle East*. London: Curzon Press.

Lippard, L. (1990). *Mixed blessings: Art in a multicultural America*. New York: Pantheon.

Lippard, L. (1995). *The pink glass swan: Selected feminist essays on art*. New York: New Press.

Lowenfield, V. (1987). *Creative and mental growth*. New York: Macmillan.

Lutz, T. (1997). The limit of Europeanness: Immigrant women in Europe. *Feminist Review, 57*, 93.

Maddrell, P. (1988). *The Bedouin of the Negev*. London: British Library.

Magos, M. (2012). Visual structures of images of employment: Images as a way to access visions of self-fulfillment in unemployed at risk young women. In E. Huss, L. Kacen, & E. Hirshen (Eds.), *Creating research, researching creations* (pp. 53–67). Bialik, Israel: Ben-Gurion University Press.

Mahon, M. (2000). The visible evidence of cultural producers. *Annual Review of Anthropology, 29*, 467–492.

Maslow, A. (1970). *Motivation and personality*. New York: Harper Collins publication.

Malchiodi, C. (1998). *Understanding children's drawings*. New York: Guilford.

Malchiodi, C. A. (2007). *The art therapy sourcebook* (2nd ed.). New York: McGraw-Hill Professional.
Malchiodi, C., & Riley, S. (1996). *Supervision and related issues*. Chicago, IL: Magnolia Street.
Mason, J. (2002). *Qualitative use of visual method*. London: Sage.
Masrey, N. (2011). *Drawings of young girls who got married before the age of seventeen* (Master's thesis). Ben-Gurion University, Beer Sheva, Israel.
Masten, A. S. (2001). Ordinary magic: Resilience processes in development. *American Psychologist, 56*, 227–238.
Mathews, X. (1994). *Children and visual representation: Helping children to draw and paint in early childhood*. London: Hodder & Stoughton.
McNiff, S. (1995). *Art based research*. Retrieved from http://bjsw.oxfordjournals.org/
McNiff, S. (1998). *Trust the process: An artist's guide to letting go*. Boston, MA: Shambhala Press.
Meir, A. (1997). *As nomadism ends*. Boulder, CO: Westview Press.
Meir, A. (2005). Bedouin, the Israeli state and insurgent planning: Globalization, localization or glocalization? *Cities, 22*(3), 201–215.
Mernissi, F. (2003). The meaning of spatial boundaries. In R. Lewis & S. Mills (Eds.), *Feminist postcolonial theory: A reader* (pp. 489–502). Edinburgh, Scotland: Edinburgh University Press.
Miller, S. M. (1996). The great chain of poverty explanations. In E. Øyen, S. M. Miller, & X. Samad (Eds.), *Poverty: A global review: Handbook of international poverty research*. Oslo, Norway: Scandinavian University Press.
Mills, S. (1991). *Discourses of difference: Women's travel writing and colonialism*. London: Routledge.
Mills, S. (1997). *Discourse, the new critical idiom*. London: Routledge Press.
Mohanty, C. T. (2003). Under western eyes: Feminist scholarship and colonial discourses. In R. Lewis & S. Mills (Eds.), *Feminist postcolonial theory: A reader* (pp. 71–92). Edinburgh: Edinburgh University Press.
Moon, B. (2000). *Ethical issues in art therapy*. Springfield, IL: Charles C. Thomas.
Moon, B. L. (2008). *Introduction to art therapy: Faith in the product* (2nd ed.). Springfield, IL: Charles C. Thomas.
Moon, H. (2002). *Studio art therapy*. London: Jessica Kingsley.
Moor, G. (1997). *Post-colonial theory: Contexts, practices, politics*. New York: Verso.
Motzafi-Heller, P. (2000). Reading Arab feminist discourses: Hagar. *International Social Science Review, 1*(2), 63–91.
Moustakas, C. (1994). *Phenomenological research methods*. Thousand Oaks, CA: Sage.
Mullen, C. (2003). A self-fashioned gallery of aesthetic practice. *Qualitative Inquiry, 9*(2), 165–82.
Naasr, S. H. (2002). *The heart of Islam*. San Francisco, CA: HarperCollins.
Naryan U. (1995). Mail-order brides: Immigrant women, domestic violence and immigration law. *Hypatia: A Journal of Feminist Philosophy, 10*(1), 104–109.
Nelson, K., & Fivush, R. (2004). The emergence of autobiographical memory: A social cultural developmental theory. *Psychological Review, 111*(2), 486–513.

Nuremberg, M. (1966). *Dynamically oriented art therapy*. New York: Grune & Stratton.
Nuttman-Shwartz, O., Huss, E., & Altman A. (2010). The experience of forced relocation as expressed in children's drawings. *Clinical Social Work, 38*(4), 397–407.
O'Callaghan, C. (2008). Object perception: Vision and audition. *Philosophy Compass, 3*(4), 803–829.
Ong, A. (2003). State versus Islam: Maley Families: Women's bodies and the body politic of Malaysia. In R. Lewis & S. Mill (Eds.), *Feminist postcolonial theory* (pp. 381–412). Edinburgh, Scotland: Edinburgh University Press.
Patton, M. (1987). *How to use qualitative methods in evaluation*. Thousand Oaks, CA: Sage.
Perez, H. (2001). My skin is my only protection. *Notes on the Bedouin, 34,* 25–31.
Pink, S. (2001). *Doing visual ethnography*. London: Sage.
Pink, S., & Kurti, L. (2004). *Working images: Visual research and representation in ethnography*. London: Routledge.
Piquemal, N. (2005). Hear the silenced voices and make that relationship: Issues of relational ethics in aboriginal contexts. In I. Abu-Saad & D. Champagne (Eds.), *Indigenous education and empowerment: International perspectives* (pp. 27–42). Lanham, MD: Altamira Press.
Pizarro, J. (2004). The efficacy of art and writing therapy: Increasing positive mental health outcomes and participant retention after exposure to traumatic experience. *Art Therapy: Journal of the American Art Association, 21*(1), 5–12.
Porat, H. (2009). *The Bedouin in the Negev between nomadism and sedentraizaiton, 1948–1973*. Ben-Gurion University, Israel: Negev Center for Development.
Razin, E., & Hasson, F. (1994). Urban-rural boundary conflicts: The reshaping of Israel's rural map. *Journal of Rural Studies, 10*(1), 47–59.
Relton, B. (2005). *Quest: Gypsy identity*. Lanham, MD: Altamira Press.
Rhyne, J. (1991). *The gestalt art experience: Patterns that connect*. Chicago, IL: Magnolia St.
Ried, P. (1993). Poor women in psychological research: Shut up and shut out. *Psychology of Women Quarterly, 17,* 133–150.
Riley, S. (1997). Social constructivism: The narrative approach and clinical art therapy. *Journal of the American Art Therapy Association, 14*(4), 282–284.
Robinson, M. (2000). *Talkin' up to the white woman: Indigenous women and feminism*. St. Lucia, Queensland: University of Queensland Press.
Rogers, N. (1993). *Expressive arts as healing*. Palo Alto, CA: Science and Behavior Books.
Rosal, M. (2001). Cognitive behavioral art therapy. In J. Rubin (Ed.), *Approaches to art therapy* (pp. 210–225). Philadelphia, PA: Brunner-Mazel.
Rose, G. (1988). *Visual methodologies*. London: Sage.
Rosenthal, G. (1993). Reconstruction of life stories: Principles of selection in generating stories for narrative biographical interviews. In R. Josselson & A. Lieblich (Eds.), *The narrative study of lives* (pp. 59–91). Newbury Park, CA: Sage.
Rubin, J. (1999). *Art therapy, an introduction*. Philadelphia. PA: Brunner-Mazel.

Rubin, J. (2001). *Approaches to art therapy*. Philadelphia, PA: Brunner–Mazel.
Runyan, A., & Peterson, S. (2009). *Global gender issues in the new millennium*. Boulder, CO: Westview Press.
Sabbagh, S. (1997). *Arab women*. Brookline, MA: Olive Branch Press.
Sadan, E. (1999). *Empowerment and community planning*. Kibbutz Meuchad, Israel: Kibbutz Meuchad. (Hebrew)
Samach, A. (2010). *Comparison of children's drawings from recognized and from unrecognized villages* (Master's thesis). Ben-Gurion University, Beer Sheva, Israel.
Sarasema, T. (2003). Bereavement and the healing power of arts and writing. *Qualitative Inquiry, 9*(4), 603–621.
Sarid, O., & Huss, E. (2010). Trauma and acute stress disorder: A comparison between cognitive behavioral intervention and art therapy. *The Arts in Psychotherapy, 37*(1), 1–8.
Saulnier, C. (1996). *Feminist theories and social work*. New York: Haworth Press.
Save, I., & Nuutinen, K. (2003). At the meeting place of word and picture: Between art and inquiry. *Qualitative Inquiry, 9*(4), 515–535.
Schaverien, J. (1999). *The revealing image: Analytical art psychotherapy in theory and in practice*. London: Routledge.
Schechter, S. (2012). *Images of death* (Master's thesis). Ben-Gurion University, Beer Sheva, Israel.
Schwartz, N. (1996). Art as healing: Observer, process, and product. *Art Therapy: Journal of the American Art Therapy Association, 13*(4), 244–251.
Sclater, D. (2003). The arts and narrative research. *Qualitative Inquiry, 9*(4), 621–625.
Segel-Englich, D., Kaufman, R., & Huss, E. (2011). Transitions in first-year students' initial practice orientations. *Journal of Social Work Education, 41*(6), 146–149.
Selva, P. (2006). Emotional processing in the treatment of psychosomatic disorders. *Journal of Clinical Psychology, 62*(5), 539–550.
Shank, M. (2005). Transforming social justice: Redefining the movement: Art activism. *Seattle Journal for Social Justice, 3*, 531–535.
Shohat, E. (1995). *Talking visual multicultural feminism in a transitional age*. New York: New Museum of Contemporary Art Press.
Silver, R. (2001). *Art as language access to thoughts and emotions through stimulus drawings*. Philadelphia, PA: Brunner-Mazel.
Silver, R. (2005). *Aggression and depression assessed through art*. New York: Brunner-Routledge.
Silverman, D. (2000). *Doing qualitative research: A practical handbook*. London: Sage.
Silverstone, L. (1993). *Art therapy the person centered way*. Philadelphia, PA: Jessica Kingsley.
Simmons, H., & Hicks, J. (2006). Opening doors: Using the creative arts in learning and teaching. *Arts and Humanities in Higher Education, 5*, 77–79.
Skaif, S., & Huet, V. (Eds.). (1998). *Art psychotherapy groups: Between pictures and groups*. London: Routledge.
Slater, N., & Al-Krenawi, A. (2004). *Bedouin Arab children use visual art as a response to the destruction of their homes in unrecognized villages*. Beer

Sheva, Israel: Ben-Gurion University of the Negev, The Center for Bedouin Studies and Development.

Smith, D. (2002). Institutional ethnography. In T. May (Ed.), *Qualitative research in action* (pp. 17–53). London: Sage.

Sofie, B., & Solvig, E. (2000). Turkish migrant women encountering health care in Stockholm: A qualitative study of somatization and illness meaning. *Culture, Medicine, and Psychiatry, 24*(4), 431–452.

Soja, E. W. (1989). *Postmodern geographies: The reassertion of space in critical social theory.* London: Verso.

Spaniol, S., & Bluebird, G. (2002). Creative partnerships, people with psychiatric disabilities and art therapists in dialogue. *Arts in Psychotherapy, 29,* 107–114.

Speiser, V., & Speiser, P. (2007). An art approach to working with conflict. *Journal of Humanistic Psychology, 47*(3), 361–366.

Spindler, G. (1997). Transmission of culture. In G. Spindler (Ed.), *Education and cultural: Anthropological approaches* (pp. 273–279). New York: Rinehart & Winston.

Spivak, G. C. (1987). *In other worlds: Essays in cultural politics.* New York: Methuen.

Spivak, G. C. (1990). *The post-colonial critic: Interviews, strategies, dialogues.* London: Routledge.

Spivak, G. C. (1996). Interview with Spivak: Subaltern talk concerning Sati. In D. Landry & G. M. MacLean (Eds.), *The Spivak Reader* (pp. 287–308). New York: Routledge.

Spivak, G. C., & Guha, R. (Eds.). (1988). *Selected subaltern studies.* New York: Oxford University Press.

Statistical Year Book of the Negev Bedoum. (1986). Jerusalem: Ben Gurion University.

Stillerman S. (2012). *Studio art group in a community rehabilitation center for people with mental health problems.* Ben Gurion Univeristy Dept. of Social Work, Ber-Sheva, Israel.

Steinberg, S., & Bar-On, D. (2002). An analysis of the group process in encounters between Jews and Palestinians using a typology for discourse classification. *Pergamon, 26,* 199–214.

Suad, J. (1997). Gender and family in the Arab world. In S. Sabbagh (Ed.), *Arab Women* (pp. 194–203). Northampton, MA: Olive Branch Press.

Sue, D. (1996). *Theory of multicultural counseling and therapy.* New York: Brooks Cole.

Sullivan, G. (2001). Artistic thinking as trans-cognitive practice: A reconciliation of the process–product dichotomy. *Visual Arts Research, 27*(1), 2–12.

Tal, S. (1980). The embroidered dress of the Bedouin women in the Negev. *Bedouin Studies Magazine, 30,* 15–25.

Tal, S. (1995). *The Bedouin women in the Negev in time of changes.* Kibbutz Lahav, the Negev, Israel: Joe Alon Center for Bedouin Culture. [Hebrew]

Talwar, S. (2007). Accessing traumatic memory through art making: An art therapy trauma protocol (ATTP). *The Arts in Psychotherapy, 34*(1), 22–35.

Taylor, J. Gilligan, C., & Sullivan, A. (1995). *Between voice and silence: Women and girls, race and relationship.* Cambridge, MA: Harvard University Press.

Third Eye Foundation. (n.d.). Retrieved from http://thirdeye2005.blogspot.com/.
Thompson, L. (2005). *The mind and heart of the negotiator* (3rd ed.). Upper Saddle River, NJ: Pearson Education.
Tsederboim, E. (2012). Self portraits as auto ethnography. In E. Huss, L. Kacen, & E. Hirshen (Eds.), *Creating research, researching creations* (pp. 221–249). Bialik, Israel: Ben-Gurion University Press. [Hebrew]
Tuhiwai-Smith, L. (1999). *Decolonizing methodologies: Research and indigenous peoples*. London: Zed.
van der Kolk, B. A., Hopper, J., & Osterman, J. (2001). Exploring the nature of traumatic memories: Combining clinical knowledge with laboratory methods. *Journal of Aggression, Maltreatment, and Trauma, 4*(2), 9–31.
van Kleef, G. A., De Dreu, C. K. W., & Manstead, A. S. R. (2004). The interpersonal effects of emotions in negotiations: A motivated information processing approach. *Journal of Personality and Social Psychology, 87*, 510–528.
Vrielynck, N., & Philippot, P. (2008). Regulating emotion during imaginal exposure to social anxiety: Impact of the specificity of information processing. *Journal of Behavior Therapy and Experimental Psychiatry, 40*(2), 274–282.
Wadeson, H. (2002). The anti-assessment devil's advocate. *Art Therapy: Journal of the American Art Therapy Association, 19*, 168–170.
Waller D. (1993). *Group interactive art therapy*. New York: Routledge.
Wang, C., & Burris, M. (1994). Empowerment through photo-novella. *Health Education Quarterly, 21*, 172–185.
Warren, B. (2008). *Using the creative arts in therapy and healthcare*. New York: Routledge.
Weiss, I., & Kaufman, R. (2006). Educating for social action: An evaluation of the impact of a fieldwork training program. *Journal of Policy Practice, 5*(1), 5–30.
Willmott, H. (2000). Death-so what? Sociology, sequestration, and emancipation. *The Sociological Review, 48*, 649–665.
Williams, G., & Wood, M. (1984). *Developmental art therapy*. Chicago, IL: Pro-Ed.
Wilson, L. (2001). Symbolism and art therapy. In J. A. Rubin (Ed.), *Approaches to art therapy: Theory and technique* (pp. 40–53). Philadelphia, PA: Brunner-Mazel.
Winnicott, D. (1958). *Collected papers: Through pediatrics to psychoanalysis*. London: Tavistock.
Wolf, M. (1992). *A thrice told tale: Feminism, postmodernism, and ethnographic responsibility*. Stanford, CA: Stanford University Press.
Wolfgang, G. (2006). The ego-psychological fallacy: A note on the birth of the meaning out of a symbol. *Journal of Jungian Theory and Practice, 7*(2), 53–60.
Yamini, M. (1996). *Feminism and Islam*. London: Garnet.
Yin, R. (1993). *Applications of case study research*. Newbury Park, CA: Sage.
Zeligman, T., & Soloman, R. (2004). *Introduction to incest: There is no truth and no mercy and no pity*. Tel Aviv, Israel: Tel Aviv University Press (Hebrew).
Zelizer, C. (2003). The role of artistic processes in peacebuilding in Bosnia-Herzegovina. *Peace and Conflict Studies, 10*(2), 62–75.

Index

aesthetic organization of images, 75–79
ant imagery, 40
art therapy and social theory: overview, 7, 73–75, 113; aesthetics of defining problems and solutions from cultural perspective, 75–79; art as social change, 3–4; hybrid perspectives of images within art therapy, 79–84; and social perspectives on image use in research, 51
art therapy, social context and methodology: overview, 7; mapping and symbolizing pain, 88–89; social context and strengths-based approach to images, 90–93; and socially contextualized solutions, 89–90; therapeutic potential of images, 85–88

Bedouin culture: and aesthetic organization of images, 75–76; and collectivist values, 11–12; transition of, 14–16; use of images within, 13–14; women and transition of, 16–17; women within, 12–13
Bedouin women's images, case study methodology: overview, 5, 19–20; data sources, 22; and ethical considerations, 23–25; image analysis, 22–23; and qualitative research validation, 23; research questions, 20; research strategy, 20–21; women's interactions with art, 21–22
Bedouin women's images, case study social context: overview, 5, 9, 11, 114; and global context for impoverished women, 18; traditional Bedouin culture and collectivist values, 11–12; transition of Bedouin culture, 14–16; use of images within traditional Bedouin culture, 13–14; women and shifting modes of visual self-expression, 17–18; women and transition of Bedouin culture, 16–17; women within traditional Bedouin culture, 12–13. *See also* group empowerment and action
Bedouin women's images, content: overview, 5–6, 36–37; inside spaces (houses), 28–30; outside spaces and mobility, 26–28; and relationship to Jewish state, 35–36; shifting spaces between Bedouin women and men, 33–35; shifting spaces between children and adults, 31–33; social analysis of, 36–37; and wish for education, 30–31
birds as symbols of pain, 40
black imagery: black clouds, 34, 38–39; and hybrid cultural realities, 58; and indirect expression of social taboos, 56, 100, 101
blue imagery, 54–55
body part imagery, 41–42
box imagery, 57

call to prayer, 1
calligraphy, 13–14, 42–43, 76
carpet imagery, 14, 76–77
challenging social narratives, 98–99
challenging verbal narratives, 52–53
children: cognition and aesthetic

organization of images, 76–77, 78–79; images and coping mechanisms, 90–92
class struggle, 53
clay crafts, 13–14
clothing imagery, 33–35
cognition: and aesthetic organization of images, 76–77, 78–79; and image construction, 2; and images as pain symbols, 55; and indirect expression of social taboos, 57–58, 70
collectivism: and Bedouin values, 12, 13; and cultural meaning of images, 65, 79; and cultural transition of Bedouin in Israel, 14–16
colored coat image analysis, 69, 72, 82–83
communication: direct confrontation with power-holders, 110–12; empathy encouragement between different groups, 107–9; and indirect negotiation of power, 103–5; and postviolence forgiveness, 109–10; of similarities and differences within conflicting groups, 106
community art and existing power structures, 3–4
compositional elements of Bedouin women's images: overview, 6; embodied symbols, 41–42; group definition of content, 44–47; images as narrative triggers, 43; mapping experience into space, 38–39; metonyms and wishes, 39–40; resistance to lack of spaces, 39; symbols of pain, 40–41; traditional versus Western symbols, 42–43; verbal and visual information gaps, 43–44
conflict negotiation: overview, 8; communication of similarities and differences within conflicting groups, 106; and direct confrontation with power-holders, 110–12; empathy encouragement between different groups, 107–9; and indirect negotiation of power and communication, 103–5; and postviolence forgiveness, 109–10; and women in traditional Bedouin culture, 12–13
content: composition and content analysis of images, 68; form and content analyses, 49–50, 51–52; group definition of content, 44–47. *See also* Bedouin women's images, content
creating and choosing images, research methodology, 66–67
cultural perspectives: art therapy and social theory, 75–79; cultural connotations of images, 64; and hybrid perspectives of images within art therapy, 79–84; images and hybrid cultural realities, 58–59; and social construction of images, 2–3
cultural transition: and Bedouin in Israel, 14–16; and Bedouin women, 16–17; and shifting spaces between Bedouin women and men, 33–35; and shifting spaces between children and adults, 31–32; and shifts in visual self-expression, 17–18; and social perspectives on image use in research, 6–7, 49–50, 51–52

definition of images within research, 64–66
discourse image analysis, 68
driver's licenses, 26–27

education, 30–31
El-Abed Bedouin, 11
embodied symbols and Bedouin women's images, 41–42
embroidery, 13–14, 17, 18, 76, 99–100
emotions: emotional response to images, 2; and images as pain symbols, 54–56
empathy encouragement between different groups, 107–9
empowerment, 46–47
envisaging solutions, 60–61
ethical considerations, Bedouin women's images research, 23–25

fish imagery, 40, 45
flow and art therapy, 85–88
form and content analyses, 49–50, 51–52

gender segregation: and Bedouin in Israel, 16–17, 33; genograms and images as narrative triggers, 59–60; and traditional cultures, 12–13
genograms, 59–60, 66, 80–81
global context for impoverished women, 18
globalization and hybrid perspectives of images within art therapy, 81
group definition of content, 44–47, 59–60
group empowerment and action: overview, 7, 94–96; art enrichment programs and group goals, 21; and challenging social narratives, 98–99; and group exhibition, 97–98; and indirect challenges of dominant narratives, 99–102; individual images within the group, 96–97

hadg carpets, 14
hands imagery, 57, 100–101
heart symbol, 41
"high context" and collectivist culture, 12
hole imagery, 57
house imagery: black circle, 44; and children's cognition, 77; and conflicting groups, 106; and image explanations, 67; and inside spaces, 28–30, 36; and spatial mapping, 38
Hum Ran Bedouin, 11
hybrid cultural realities, 58–59
hybrid perspectives of images within art therapy, 79–84

identity and image analysis, 70–71
image analysis and explanations, 22–23, 67–69
image-based workshops: human responses to, 2; and relations with Bedouin women, 1–2; research methodology, 20–21
image use in social research and practice, 49–50
images: construction of and universal development stages, 2; and indirect negotiation of power and communication, 61–62, 103–5; as narrative triggers, 43, 59–60; as social constructs, 2–3; and traditional Bedouin culture, 13–14

images and research methodology, 63–72; overview, 7, 63; image definitions, 64–66; and image explanations, 67; observation of creating or choosing images as data, 66–67, 69–70; and position of images within research, 69–72; and researcher analysis of images, 22–23, 67–69. *See also* art therapy and social theory; social perspectives on image use in research
indirect challenges of dominant narratives, 99–102
indirect conflict negotiation, 12–13, 61–62, 103–5
indirect expression of social taboos, 56–58
individual images within groups, 96–97
information gaps, verbal and visual information gaps, 43–44
inside spaces (houses), 28–30
invisibility of Bedouin society in Israel, 15–16

Jewish state relationships, 35–36
Joseph's colored coat image analysis, 69, 72, 82–83

lack of space and Bedouin women's images, 39
land conflicts, 15, 16
language and image studies, 3, 4
"lost" children, 31–33, 38

mapping and symbolizing pain, 88–89
mapping experience into space: and challenging verbal narratives, 52–53; compositional elements of Bedouin women's images, 38–39
material types: and image creation, 65–66; and observation of image creation, 66–67
men, shifting spaces between Bedouin women and men, 33–35
metonyms and wishes, 39–40
mobility, outside spaces and mobility, 26–28
mother-in-law/daughter-in-law relationships, 17
Muezzin's call to prayer, 1

narratives: challenging social narratives, 98–99; challenging verbal narratives, 52–53; and image explanations, 67; images as narrative triggers, 59–60; indirect challenges to dominant narratives, 99–102; narrative triggers and Bedouin women's images, 43
nature: and culturally acceptable expressions of emotion, 40–41; traditional versus Western symbols, 42–43
nomadism: and cultural transition of Bedouin in Israel, 14–16; and sheep and tent imagery, 27, 28
non-verbal images as pain symbols, 54–56

observation of creating or choosing images, 66–67
oral traditions in Bedouin culture, 13–14
orange imagery, 91
outside spaces and mobility, 26–28

pain symbols: compositional elements of Bedouin women's images, 40–41; mapping and symbolizing pain, 88–89; and social perspectives on image use in research, 54–56
phenomenological image analysis, 22–23, 51–52, 68, 81–82. *See also* art therapy and social theory; group empowerment and action
polygamy, 17, 31, 32
position of images within research, 69–72
postviolence forgiveness, 109–10
poverty: houses and inside space imagery, 28–30; and shifting spaces between Bedouin women and men, 33–35; and shifting spaces between children and adults, 31–33; wish for education and Bedouin women's images, 30–31
power structures: Bedouin women's images case study overview, 19–20; destabilization of, 3–4; direct confrontation of, 110–12; and ethics of art therapy research, 24–25; gender segregation and traditional cultures, 12–13; indirect negotiation with, 61–62, 103–5; and shifting spaces between Bedouin women and men, 33–35; women and group definitions of content, 46–47. *See also* conflict negotiation; group empowerment and action
privacy and ethics of art therapy research, 24
psychoanalytical image analysis, 68
pure content image analysis, 67–68

research. *See* images and research methodology; social perspectives on image use in research
resilience. *See* compositional elements of Bedouin women's images
resistance: to lack of spaces, 39; women and group definitions of content, 44–47
rope metaphor and image use in research, 63

sedentary lifestyle: and cultural transition of Bedouin in Israel, 14–16, 18; and sheep and tent imagery, 27, 28
self-portraits, 21–22
sexual self-expression, 34
sheep and tent imagery, 27, 28
social construction of images, 2–3
social context: and cultural norms, 11; and strengths-based approach to images, 90–93. *See also* Bedouin women's images, case study social context
social norms and image construction, 3
social perspectives on image use in research: overview, 6–7, 49–50, 51–52; and envisaging solutions, 60–61; and hybrid cultural realities, 58–59; images as narrative triggers, 59–60; images as pain symbols, 54–56; and indirect expression of social taboos, 56–58; and indirect negotiation with power-holders, 61–62; mapping experience into space, 52–53
social taboos: and images as pain symbols, 55; indirect expression of, 56–58
social theory. *See* art therapy and social theory

socially contextualized solutions and art therapy, 79–84, 89–90
solutions: images as envisaging solutions, 60–61; socially contextualized solutions and art therapy, 79–84, 89–90
space as political issue, 53
spatial mapping, 38–39
standing and talking imagery, 61
Sum Ran Bedouin, 11
swimming pool imagery, 26, 27–28

tent imagery, 28, 43
traditional versus Western symbols, 42–43
transformation of meaning, 59–60
trash imagery, 52–53, 96–97
trees: and envisaging solutions, 61; as personified crying image, 41; as symbols of pain, 41; and traditional versus Western symbols, 42–43; tree metaphor and role of men, 33

vase imagery, 102
verbal and visual information gaps, 43–44
verbal data and image analysis, 70–71
visualizations and researcher analysis of images, 67–69

war situations: and aesthetic organization of images, 77–78; conflict groups and postviolence forgiveness, 109–10; images and coping mechanisms, 92–93; and images as pain symbols, 55–56
weaving, 13–14, 76
Western culture and aesthetic organization of images, 76
Western versus traditional symbols, 42–43
wishes: and Bedouin women's images, 39–40; for education, 30–31; for mobility and outside spaces, 26–28
women and group definitions of content, 44–47

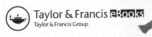